D0456561

The
Fibromyalgia
Relief
Handbook

Chet Cunningham

United Research Publishers
www.unitedresearchpubs.com

Published by United Research Publishers

Printed and bound in the United States of America

ISBN 1-887053-13-1

Library of Congress Control Number 00-131420

The information in this book is not intended to replace the advice of your physician. You should consult your doctor regarding any medical condition which concerns you. The material presented in this book is intended to inform and educate the reader with a view to making some intelligent choices in pursuing the goal of living life in a healthy, vigorous manner.

Order additional copies from:

> United Research Publishers
> P.O. Box 232344
> Encinitas CA 92023-2344

or:

> www.unitedresearchpubs.com

Full 90-day money-back guarantee if not satisfied.

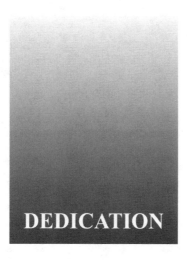

DEDICATION

This book is dedicated to Roger Neuman, who has devoted much of his life to bringing vital medical information to the public in a form that is easy to understand and to act upon. His talents have made more than ten medical problems simpler to learn about and that has made a huge difference in thousands of lives.

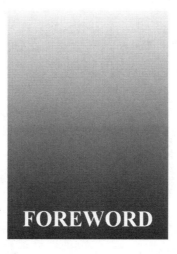

FOREWORD

A word before you begin reading this book. First, I am not a doctor. I'm a person interested in fibromyalgia. I want to learn all I can about it. That means I want it explained in easy to understand layman's language. That's the overall guideline for this book.

No complicated, obtuse or detailed medical terminology will be used without it being explained in common, ordinary English words.

Every attempt has been made to present this strange and complex group of ailments and pains and problems we call fibromyalgia in easy-to-understand explanations, terms and suggestions that we hope will help you to start to feel better.

We're all on the same level here. If I don't understand it, I can't write it so you can understand it.

Now, you're free to go ahead and dig into this fascinating, frustrating and often debilitating group of pains and problems. We hope that this book will help you to feel better, live larger, and enjoy life more. Hey, it's the only life we have.

TABLE OF CONTENTS

CHAPTER 1

WHAT IS FIBROMYALGIA?

Fibromyalgia is a serious medical problem that involves some or all of the following symptoms: intense chronic muscle pain, fatigue, headaches, sleeping problems, joint pain, numbness and tingling, irritable bowel syndrome, problems with memory and concentration, sensitivity to cold, bladder complications, depression, and a swelling sensation of the hands.

Doctors don't know what causes it: therefore it is difficult to figure out how to cure it. They do have a short name, though. They call it FibroMyalgia Syndrome, or FMS. We'll use the term as well.

These aches and pains can come almost anywhere in the body, and can include one or two or ten or twelve different areas. The pain is often what brings on other problems, especially the mental ones, and depression.

For many years, doctors had no idea what this group of problems actually was. Often FMS was passed off as a patient's imagination or just feeling "out of sorts." People who have X-rays and blood tests and other physical exams do not show any sign of what is causing the pain. It's there—and even ten years ago, doctors had no idea what was going on.

Today, some doctors still don't, so if you have fibromyalgia, be sure to find a doctor who knows about it and how to treat it.

This problem is not fatal, and most people are relieved to know what they have and that it isn't some serious bone cancer or other fatal ailment. Fibromyalgia is not consistent. You may hurt one place one day and not the next. Your symptoms may be excruciating for a few months and then almost vanish in certain parts of your body.

The problem with FMS is that it will not go away. Quite simply put, there is no cure for fibromyalgia. In many cases the symptoms will interfere with your work, your pleasure, even your sleeping. Research is continuing to find a cause. Much work must be done before effective treatment is found to go after the cause and not just to reduce the symptoms.

FMS is most common in middle-aged women from 30 to 50 years of age. Seven to ten million Americans suffer to some degree with FMS. Some young children have it, and some elderly, but most of the cases are in the 30-50 year range of women. Some experts say that more than fifty women have the problem to every case of a man with it. That still means that 20,000 men will have fibromyalgia. Others in the field say they are now finding that twenty-five percent of their patients with FMS are men. They say this may be due to better diagnosis of men patients.

One point here to understand. FMS is not the same as arthritis. Arthritis is a problem with the immune system attacking the joints rather than protecting them. The joints themselves are the victims, and not the muscles or tendons around the joints. It may seem like your joints hurt with FMS, but in reality it is the soft muscles and tissues around the joint that are causing the pain.

The hurt can feel much the same, and in many cases the patient limits the use of the arm or leg, or cuts down on physical activity so the leg won't hurt as much. We'll discuss this later when we get into exercise. For right now, exercise will help, rather than hurt your FMS.

HOW CAN YOU TELL IF YOU HAVE FIBROMYALGIA?

The best diagnostic tool the doctors have so far is the palpation test. This simply means the doctor will press with his fingers on various parts of your body. Over the years, doctors have learned where to find these tender points. They pinpoint tender areas in specific locations.

Generally your doctor will take a complete personal and family history to rule out other health problems. The pressure tests are done on eighteen tender points on the body. If the pain has been there for three months, and the doctor finds sensitivity in eleven of the eighteen points, it's probable that the patient has fibromyalgia.

Where are these tender points? They always come in pairs. There are two on the throat about where the carotid arteries are situated. Two more are located below the clavicle about two inches and about four inches apart. Two more are found on the inside of the front of the leg and just above the knee.

On the back, there are two tender points on the upper neck, two more about half way down from neck to the shoulder, and two more about four inches below the shoulder points in the back.

The back of the elbow finds another point on each arm. Two more are located in the lower back about four inches below the waist, and the last two are on the back of the outside of the hips.

WHAT ARE THE SYMPTOMS OF FMS?

Pain in soft tissue is a primary symptom. This pain might be burning, gnawing, radiating, shooting, or just a dull ache. These pains can be severe or mild, but they are felt deep inside the muscle, ligament and tendons. Joint pain may also be present.

When you hurt, the pain might be in your hips, thighs, knees, legs, buttocks, neck, elbows, wrists arms, shoulders, back, chest, feet or ankles. You might hurt in one or all of these places.

Your doctor will ask you about other symptoms. These are the primary ailments that FMS can produce:

FATIGUE: This is one of the most common problems associated with FMS. You might get over your bad night's sleep by noon, but by afternoon you will get so tired and slow and even sleepy that it will be hard to do your work. The problem worsens as the afternoon wears on. Fatigue all day can lead to total exhaustion at quitting time, but then chances are a real restful sleep will not be possible.

POOR SLEEP SYNDROME: All but ten percent of FMS sufferers have some type of sleep problem. It could be difficulty falling asleep, waking up several times each night, tossing all night without sleep, waking up early in the morning and not being able to get back to sleep. Or it could be insomnia without the ability to get to sleep.

Some FMS patients get to sleep and think they are getting restful sleep, but in reality they are not. Their sleep is disturbed, and not the deep restorative type needed. Nobody knows why this happens. Some experts say that sleep problems may be part of the cause of muscle pain. The muscles don't get their usual regenerative rest period and react the next day with pain.

HEADACHES: Surveys show that about forty percent of those with FMS have headaches at least once a day. Many of these are severe. Patients report that tension headaches usually start with strain or tightness in the upper neck, often from muscle tightness.

Migraine headaches happen, but usually at no higher rate than for people without FMS.

JOINT PAIN: FMS can lead to pain in hands, elbows, neck, wrists, feet, ankles, knees, hips and the chest wall. We call this joint pain, but the pain is usually felt over the joint area and is not associated with the joint. Doctors tell us that this pain often happens where the tendon attaches to the bone. If you think you have tendinitis after some strenuous activity, use the normal tendinitis treatments of ice, rest, aspirin or cortisone. If the problem does not respond to those treatments, it could be FMS and not tendinitis.

TINGLING AND NUMBNESS: These neurological symptoms show up in arms and legs of only a quarter of the people who have FMS. Those who have it say it makes their hands feel swollen and clumsy. We don't know what causes these problems and there is no special treatment.

IRRITABLE BOWEL SYNDROME: About a third of FMS patients have some of the problems associated with an irritable bowel. These include bloating, gas, abdominal pain, diarrhea, constipation and various other digestive disorders. Correct diet, prescriptions and over-the-counter remedies can usually handle these problems. Consult your doctor or a gastroenterologist.

POSSIBLE SWELLING: Some FMS patients say they feel swelling of their ankles, feet and hands. The problem is that usually there is no actual swelling, only the feeling of swelling. If there is actual swelling, it may be the result of some other problem such as arthritis, phlebitis or a hormonal imbalance.

CHEST WALL PAIN: Pain in the chest wall is important for FMS patients because it could be a heart problem. A third of FMS patients report this type of pain. Most who are tested show no heart problems. Another indication that this pain is in the chest wall is when the patient reports tenderness when the chest is palpated.

This fibromyalgia symptom can be treated with therapy and medication to control the pain. Your doctor will prescribe.

SENSITIVE TO COLD: Some forty percent of people with FMS have trouble with cold hands. Small blood vessels in the hands over-react to cold temperatures and begin to spasm. The result can be the fingers and hand changing colors from white to blue and then red. Along with it can come stinging, pain, numbness and tingling. See your doctor. Warming the affected hand can produce temporary relief.

CONCENTRATION AND MEMORY: A quarter of the people

with FMS report memory and concentration problems. A person may go to a room and forget why he or she went there. Sometimes the right words to complete a sentence won't come. Others say they sometimes have trouble completing a project or reading.

Other symptoms of fibromyalgia include:

- Chronic aching
- Stiffness
- Anxiety
- Depression
- Dizziness, palpitations
- Irritable bladder
- Muscular twitching
- Sensitive skin
- Dry eyes and mouth
- Frequent changes in eye prescriptions
- Impaired coordination
- Urinary frequency
- Restless leg syndrome
- Painful menstrual cramps

Some people with FMS say it's hard to make others understand how they feel. They say: Think back to the last time you had the flu. Every muscle in your body ached and you felt totally drained of energy. This describes how many people with FMS feel. Only it doesn't go away in a week or two the way the flu does.

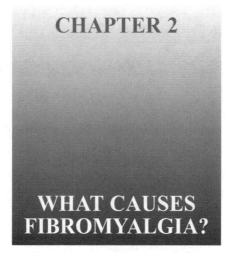

CHAPTER 2

WHAT CAUSES FIBROMYALGIA?

For every action, there is a reaction. For every cause there is an effect. For every disease or clinical disorder, there is a cause.

Yes, but finding that cause of a disease or a clinical disorder is a huge task, and one not easily satisfied. Usually there must be concrete proof, something that will show on an X-ray or a CAT scan or an MRI, or in an overwhelming statistical report of double-blind clinical tests.

Right now, there is no proof of what causes fibromyalgia. There are a batch of theories and speculations, and half-proven treatments that could indicate a cause. We don't even know if there is one cause, or a variety of causes that produce the variety of bodily problems created in the FM Syndrome.

So, where does that leave us? We take a long hard look at the evidence that the best in the field have turned up, reported, and promoted. We let the experts in this area evaluate them and take what shakes down.

Right now, early in the new millenium (of the year 2000), there is no proven cure for FMS.

However there is progress in trying to find the "why" behind this serious group of symptoms. Here are some of the theories about what causes FMS. Some of these are based on psychological reasons, others delve into chemical and biological potential causes. We'll look at these one at a time:

STRESS

There is strong support for the idea that FMS is basically a psychosocial disorder. That it is partly the result of our fast-paced and highly competitive lifestyle. The idea is that stress alters some element in the brain that results in some or all of the various symptoms of fibromyalgia.

These supporters point out that FMS is more prevalent in our highly competitive Western society than in under-developed countries. Most developed countries report FMS. While most of the third world countries don't report any FMS, this does not mean that it is not present in some form.

Frustration may be an important factor. People with FMS show a much higher rate of frustration than those with other medical problems. This may be a result of the FMS and not the cause, since people who can't sleep properly, have aches and pains all over their bodies and feel tired all of the time, naturally would be more frustrated at life's little problems than individuals who are feeling good.

Some say that the body simply can't function normally when it's under intense stress. There is a chance that the autonomic nervous system does not work properly under continued stress. Over long periods of stress, the body seems to interrupt the natural physiological process of energy production. This and other factors could weaken the body's immune system until the body reacts with some of the various problems of fibromyalgia.

DEPRESSION

Most researchers working on the cause of FMS now say that depression probably isn't a contributing factor in the cause of FMS.

They say that only about thirty percent of FMS individuals are seriously depressed. The theory now is that this depression may be the result of the FMS and not the cause. The depression often comes after the onset of FMS and not before.

TRAUMATIC EXPERIENCES

There is a growing belief that long lasting emotional traumatic experiences may have a direct bearing on FMS. One doctor reports that almost one hundred percent of his fibromyalgia patients have gone through a long period of emotional trauma. This might have been a divorce, a car accident, some long debilitating illness, child abuse, or growing up in a dysfunctional family environment.

The theory here is that the traumatic events in themselves did not cause the FMS, but they may have triggered the attacks. The trauma may have provoked some deep-seated physiological abnormality that had been latent in the individual. Now, with this prodding, the FMS rears up and the symptoms appear.

Once the FMS shows itself, it can affect the patient to launch other FMS problems. Pain may cause a person to cut down on activity, and that can result in anxiety and stress and even depression.

CHRONIC FATIGUE

Fatigue is the most common symptom of people with FMS.

Many describe the feeling as the same as when they have the flu. A total drain of energy and the desire to do absolutely nothing but rest. The severity of fatigue varies with different individuals. For some it is mild, while in others it is so severe that they are totally incapacitated. For these severe cases, fatigue becomes the worst problem of FMS, even more than the pain in various parts of the body.

Those persons with serious chronic fatigue are often beset by the problem of not getting enough or the right kind of sleep, which only makes the fatigue factor worse.

DISRUPTION OF DEEP SLEEP

Almost all who suffer from some symptoms of FMS have some type of sleep disorder. This often is a disruption of deep sleep—where the most restorative benefits of sleep come.

Studies in sleep labs have shown that the tested FMS patients had little trouble falling asleep, but were interrupted numerous times by sudden bursts of brain activity. Researchers said these brain activities were much the same as awake-brain functioning.

With reduced deep sleep, the patient also produces less growth hormone, which is vital in healthy muscles and soft tissue. So the lack of deep sleep can be the cause of additional FMS problems.

Many of those with FMS wake up in the morning feeling like they didn't get a minute of good sleep. They are tired and not refreshed. This is sometimes called nonrestorative sleep. Such a problem will mean that muscles that were hurting the day before did not get enough rest and rejuvenation, and they will also hurt again the next day.

Some fibromyalgia patients have a sleep disorder called Alpha-EEG. Other problems with sleeping include nighttime jerking of arms and legs, sleep apnea, restless leg syndrome and teeth grinding.

While sleep disorders may not be a basic cause of FMS, they can certainly contribute to the problem and beget new symptoms.

GROWTH HORMONE DEFICIENCY

As noted in the material above, the disruption of deep sleep impairs the production of growth hormone. This hormone has a lot to do with restoring damaged and fatigued muscles. If these fibers can't be refreshed during sleep, as they normally would be, it creates a continuing problem for pain in any of the eighteen tender points.

LOW LEVELS OF MAGNESIUM, PHOSPHATE, AND OXYGEN SUBSTRATE

Researchers in various areas are now reporting that FMS patients are showing deficiencies in at least three substances. These three are magnesium, phosphate, and oxygen substrate. All are essential for the body to produce energy. High levels of these three mean that the body can continue healthy cell respiration and the production of biological energy.

Withdraw these elements and there is an inability of the body to utilize oxygen for muscle energy. The result? In many FMS people it will produce fatigue—and soon depression.

SEROTONIN LEVEL

Serotonin is a chemical in the brain. Anxiety, depression and anger all cause stress. That stress helps to deplete the brain chemical serotonin. When that happens, it elevates the substance called P. When this substance P is too high it makes the pain you feel much more intense. The increased pain causes anxiety, depression and anger, which produces stress. That stress helps to deplete the brain chemical serotonin.

Which just cycles around again, regenerating the pain and the anxiety and the stress all over again.

Serotonin can't yet be measured in the brain, so it is checked in the spinal fluid where its metabolic by-product 5-HIAA collects.

People with FMS have less of the serotonin by-product than normal individuals. This lack may be because the emotional response of the person to stress uses up some of it. Control the stress and you control the level of serotonin.

THE INHERITANCE FACTOR

More and more researchers today feel that the tendency to develop FMS is inherited. An Ohio State study says that this inheritance will affect only half the children of a fibromyalgia patient.

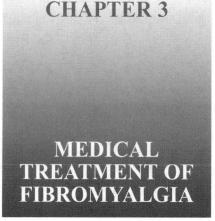

CHAPTER 3

MEDICAL TREATMENT OF FIBROMYALGIA

Once you have been diagnosed as having fibromyalgia, the first question you may have is: "How can I treat this problem?"

MOIST HEAT

Many doctors will advise you to give moist heat a try. Some of you may have used dry heating pads to moderate your pain. They work to a degree. But moist heat in the form of a shower, whirlpool, warm swimming pool, bath or hot towel works lots better.

Soak in a shower? You bet. Get a plastic chair and put it in the shower and sit there and aim the hot water at your main pain and let it run. As the pain moderates, you can move the showerhead around to hit other areas of your body that hurt. The hot water pouring down your back or stomach will reach many of the major pain points of fibromyalgia. Try this hot water treatment twenty minutes at a time, twice a day. Almost at once you're going to notice a difference in the pain.

Be careful in bathtubs. They are tough to get in and out of if your pain is extreme. Remember that, after a hot bath, you may be weaker than normal. Take extreme care getting in and out of a tub or a whirlpool. Help may be needed.

If you can't use a shower, tub or pool, try heating towels in hot water, wringing them out and putting them on the painful area. Change the towels as soon as they start to cool down. This takes a lot of work, but if someone helps you, it goes well.

Many doctors say that the moist heat treatments twice a day will be the most productive in reducing pain of any of the methods you might try.

So do it.

DRUG TREATMENTS

Today the basic treatment for fibromyalgia is the use of drugs to reduce pain and to help the patient get good restful sleep. Most experts say that the sleeping problems almost all FMS patients have are the major factors in creating and making worse many of the symptoms of fibromyalgia. So, many of the medications are aimed at aiding in sleeping—to get a deep sleep that will let the body refresh itself and boost the body's production of serotonin. Serotonin is a neuro-transmitter which modulates sleep and aids the immune system. The hope here is that with more sleep, the body can become healthier and moderate the pain problems.

Medications are not the only answer for the FMS patient, but they are a starting place. One of the problems with prescribing drugs is that they often only mask the pain, and do nothing to eliminate it. The use of drugs almost always has side effects. In some cases these can be worse than the problem the drug was taken for. But even with these cautions, there are always times when pain-relieving drugs are the only way to treat some fibromyalgia pain.

Before taking any drugs—for any problem—you should know what they are supposed to do and what the side effects can be. You and your doctor should evaluate the various drugs used and pick the best one for you that will do the job and have the fewest side effects.

The lack of a good night's sleep is one of the toughest problems of FMS. Experts say it may result in fatigue, headaches, and memory and concentration difficulties. Lack of restful sleep can also lead to pain and muscle atrophy. As of yet, there are no magical cures for sleep dysfunction. There are drugs that can do part of the job, and we'll look at these.

A caution here. The information concerning drugs is not in any way intended to take the place of medication prescribed by your doctor. This material is for information only. Your doctor will talk over your case, evaluate your symptoms and then prescribe for you.

Remember that using another person's medication is never a good idea. Every case of FMS is different and medications are always personalized for the individual.

Generally the problems created by drug side effects are almost always multiplied if medications are taken with caffeine or alcohol. A side effect of many medications is drowsiness. If it is listed on your prescription as a side effect, take the medication just before you go to bed. Then you can use the drowsiness to help you sleep better and it won't mess up your daytime.

Here are some of the most used drugs for FMS patients:

ANTIDEPRESSANTS

These drugs are non-addictive and given to help a patient get to sleep better and sleep longer and deeper. The mechanics of these drugs is to help the body to boost its level of serotonin These drugs have helped patients to better sleeping, but they have side effects such as daytime drowsiness, dry mouth, increased appetite and constipation.

Stay away from prescription sleeping medications and tranquilizers in the benzodiazepine group. These drugs can help sleep, but they depress deep sleep—and that can make fibromyalgia worse and not better. Other sleeping meds to avoid include valium, restoril and halcion. They also ruin your deep sleep and can be highly addictive.

The reasonable point here is to find the medication that relieves as much pain as possible with the fewest bad side effects. Usually about half the FMS patients and their doctors figure out the best medication that will do the job. The rest keep looking.

There are some newer drugs now on the market that have had some success for FMS people. Some of them treat depression by increasing the effect of serotonin. Another plus here is that many of the newer medications have fewer side effects than the traditional ones. Your doctor may combine two or more of the drugs with smaller doses each to achieve better results. The individual smaller doses also cut down on the severity of the side effects. Here are some of those newer drugs:

- Amitriptyline
- Elavil
- Clobenzaprine
- Xanax
- Paxil
- Klonopin

There are side effects with some of these drugs that include dry mouth, increased appetite, constipation and daytime drowsiness.

CORTICOSTEROIDS:

Two powerful drugs, cortisone and prednisone, may be prescribed for severe pain. The long-term use of high doses of these drugs put them in the dangerous category. Side effects from these two drugs include slow wound healing, risk of bone fracture, thinning of bones. Other long-term use can cause osteoporosis, diabetes, hypertension and even mental disturbances. These are two good medications to avoid if at all possible.

These drugs can also mean the decrease of absorption of vitamin D, and speed up the excretion of vitamin C, potassium and zinc. If you must take a corticosteroid, increase your intake of vitamins D and C, and potassium and zinc.

ACETAMINOPHEN & NSAIDS:

First the acronym. NSAID comes from the words NonSterodial Anti-Inflammatory Drug. Both of these types of drugs are prescribed by doctors for similar reasons.

Acetaminophen is better known under the trade names of

Tylenol, Liquiprin and Datril. The best known NSAIDs are Advil, Motrin and aspirin.

Both of these drugs are used for pain relief, and both do a good job. But they are not the same. Acetaminophen is an analgesic and an antipyretic. It relieves pain and lowers a fever.

NSAIDs reduce pain, reduce fever, and help reduce inflammation of tissue.

Acetaminophen is generally safe if taken as directed. However, when taken in large doses over a long period of time, it can cause problems in liver and kidney function.

The most common of the NSAIDs is aspirin, which has been around and extensively used for over a hundred years. It is a salicylate, and used to fight pain in FMS as well as for osteoarthritis, several types of rheumatism and other pains. Usually small doses are used against pain and larger doses to reduce inflammation. Aspirin is also used as a heart attack preventative.

It wasn't until the 1960s that Advil was developed, along with Indocin, Excedrin, Midol, Nuprin and Motrin.

These NSAIDs work by slowing the production of prostaglandins, hormones in the body that enhance inflammation and pain. These same prostaglandins also are vital to a lot of other bodily functions including blood pressure, coagulation, and kidney regulation.

Long term use of NSAIDs can have serious side effects that include:

- nausea
- indigestion
- cramps
- diarrhea
- constipation
- sunlight sensitivity
- confusion
- nervousness
- drowsiness
- headache
- sore throat

- high blood pressure
- swelling hands and feet
- ulcers
- weight gain
- urinary problems

So both the acetaminophens and the NSAIDs can offer good relief for the fibromyalgia person, however they should not be used in large doses over a long period of time.

Even when taking prescribed NSAIDs, there are some helpful notes to protect yourself:

- Usually take NSAIDs with food. It's best to eat half your meal, then take your pills, and then eat the rest. This protects your stomach.
- Drink at least eight ounces of water if taking the pills without food. The water protects your stomach and esophagus.
- Don't lie down for a half-hour after you take the NSAID pills with water. Gravity helps the pills pass through your esophagus.
- Always take the exact dosage your doctor prescribed.
- Pregnant or breast-feeding women should not take NSAIDs.
- Do not drink alcohol while taking NSAIDs. It increases stomach problems.
- Never combine acetaminophen with a NSAID. One or the other.
- If you are given a prescription for one or the other, tell your doctor all of the medications you are taking.
- If you are taking NSAIDs and having surgery, tell your doctor or dentist.
- Avoid driving if you take NSAIDs. The medication can cause drowsiness, confusion or dizziness.
- Limit your exposure to the sun if you take NSAIDs. They make your skin extra sensitive to the sun.

MUSCLE RELAXANTS

If your muscle pain becomes too severe, you might want to

try some muscle relaxant medication. The good thing here is that they can be used as needed. Most patients report rapid relief, but it may last for only a few hours. If they don't work for you, drop them.

The brand names of some of these relaxants include: Flexeril, Parafon, Forte, Robaxin and Soma. In some clinical tests, Flexeril was shown to be effective in 30 to 40 percent of cases. The best time to take this med is at bedtime. Here the side effects usually are not serious—with the biggest being drowsiness.

NARCOTIC MEDICATIONS

Any narcotic medications must be used with extreme caution.

For a fibromyalgia patient there is a double danger. They may reduce the pain but they also can become addictive and perpetuate the patient's inactivity. They also can amplify depression, which may already may be one of the patient's problems.

In extreme cases where nothing else will relieve the debilitating pain, narcotic medications may be needed for short periods of time.

The patient who uses narcotics for pain must then expand and increase her activity in exercise and motion to justify the pain remedy. Hopefully the increased activity will help alleviate the pain.

Another problem with narcotics is that, when used regularly, they will usually result in constipation.

ANXIETY MEDICATIONS

Just living with fibromyalgia day by day can produce anxiety. When mixed with constant pain, fatigue, depression or stress the problem becomes serious.

Some doctors prescribe Xanax for anxiety and depression. About half of fibromyalgia patients respond well to this treatment when combined with ibuprofen. For some it takes from two to four months to show the full effect. Side effects are not

serious here but there may be some decreased alertness and
some sleepiness.

RESTFUL SLEEP MEDICATIONS

If you have sleep problems, have a good long talk with your
doctor about the chance of using sleeping pills. Sometimes
they help. Sometimes they mess up the works, such as by making depression worse. Let your doctor help you decide if they
would help you and, if so, which one to try.

There are three commonly used: Elavil, Sinequan and
Flexeril.

All are prescription. Small doses may be helpful to your getting uninterrupted deep sleep.

You may want to try an over-the-counter sleep aid called
melatonin. This is a hormone that is produced in the body at
night by the pineal gland. This hormone helps to set your
brain's biological clock. It determines your body's circadian
rhythms including your sleep-wake cycle, digestive functions
and even your body temperature.

Melatonin can be purchased at heath food stores, where it
is listed as a natural supplement. As a supplement it is not reg-
ulated by the Food and Drug Administration. It has been
hyped as the best thing since strawberry jam and beneficial for
half a dozen ailments and anti-aging.

Melatonin has been helpful to some FMS patients. It has
not helped others. One research program showed that melatonin taken at night induced sleep quicker—and that sleep last-
ed longer—than did that of those who had the placebo.

There have been no double blind studies on melatonin that
have been published. There are few hard facts about it as of yet.

If you wish to try it, talk over the idea with your doctor
first, and then decide. If you use it, try a small dose at first and
keep a detailed journal of the results, as contrasted to your pre-
use experience.

Can sweat and heat be the best answer? Some studies have
shown that for those with sleep problems, good old-fashioned
sweat may be one of the solutions. They report that a good

exercise program in the afternoon that produces lots of sweat and some tired muscles will benefit the sleep process. The theory here is that this exercise raises the body temperature during the workout. This increased body temperature may linger, and allows the body to go into deeper sleep at nighttime.

The same thing may work with a twenty-minute hot bath or shower about three hours before bedtime. Again the body temperature is elevated by the hot water, and a deeper sleep is produced. The hot shower or bath will also aid in making those aching muscles feel better too, which may be part of the reason you get a deeper sleep. This idea is something to sleep on.

EXPERIMENTAL MEDICATIONS

As with any medical problem that has no scientific cause and therefore no proven method or medications for treatment, fibromyalgia has a host of "magical" cures and "hype". Let's take a look at some of them. Then you and your doctor can decide if any of them might help you.

GUAIFENESIN

Here is one of the medications that many tout as the best magical cure of the century for FMS. There are no published reports or clinical trials evaluating guaifenesin. However, many fibromyalgia patients report that they have had good results with it.

What is it? Guaifenesin is an inexpensive expectorant that is an ingredient in many over-the-counter cough remedies. It's been around for many years. It is mainly used for those with bronchial or lung problems and helps those patients to thin out the mucus so it's easier to get rid of.

Some say that, for FMS patients, the guaifenesin helps the kidneys to excrete and lower the amount of phosphate in the blood.

With a low dose, symptoms do not subside for "several months."

Any benefits that guaifenesin brings can be blocked by the presence of salicylates (aspirin) in your body. If you wish to try this substance, you'll need to eliminate salicylates from your diet. Some cosmetics and hygiene products also have salicylates in them.

If you want to try this product, talk with your doctor and go with the recommendations for your specific case. This product can't hurt you and it has almost no side effects.

DETROL FOR THE BLADDER

If you have an overactive bladder, then this relatively new drug, Detrol, recently approved by the FDA, may be of help to you.

The way to treat FMS is by concentrating on one symptom at a time. If you have urinary urgency, frequency, or incontinence, keep reading.

Detrol is a brand name for tolterodine tartrate, but you don't have to remember that. This is the first new prescription in some time for treating the overactive bladder and the three problems noted above.

Bladder problems can shut you away in your house, cut down on your social calendar, and make you miserable. Ask your doctor about it. Usual dosage is two milligrams twice a day. Patients say they have had a real drop in urination frequency.

Side effects? Not dramatic Some patients may have dry mouth, headache, constipation, indigestion or dry eyes.

NADH

Researchers at Georgetown University ran a test giving NADH to patients with chronic fatigue syndrome, which is clinically almost the same as the fatigue symptoms of FMS patients. They show that NADH given to patients produced relief from fatigue, increased strength and endurance, as well as an increase in physical and mental energy. NADH is a natural enzyme and a part of all living cells. It plays a big part in the body's energy producing capability.

There is no absolute correlation between this study and the fatigue element of FMS, but it does look favorable. Consult your doctor if you think that NADH might help your fatigue problems.

SUPER MALIC ACID

Fibromyalgia muscle pain is probably caused by low muscle-tissue oxygen pressure, according to the experts. Some of them think that malic acid may be an important factor in this pain problem. Malic acid comes from apples, apricots, plums, cherries and dried dates and figs.

In a test, volunteer FMS patients took 1,220 to 2,400 mgs of malic acid. Two days later they had greatly improved pain relief. In a continued test, when the patients discontinued the malic acid for 48 hours, they went back to their normal pain level.

Super Malic, a commercial medication, is now available. In a test, patients took 200 mg of malic acid and 50 mg of magnesium. No changes were reported in their pain by the patients. They pushed the pills up to six a day, or 1,200 mg of malic acid. Some reduction in pain was noted after a longer test period.

See your doctor about this one, but know that you should give the pills two months for a fair trial.

GROWTH HORMONE

We have seen before that serotonin helps to increase the body's production of human growth hormone. The hormone is now available in pill form, but is extremely expensive and must be obtained with a prescription. Researchers say that fibromyalgia patients with muscle pain have a lower level of human growth hormone than is normal.

However, there have been no tests with human growth hormone on FMS patients. This potential aid in fighting FMS is still in the early research stages, and much work must be done before any hint of a treatment can be developed.

OTHER WAYS TO TREAT PAIN

TENS

This is an acronym that stands for Transcutaneous Electrical Nerve Stimulation. It uses electrical impulses shot into specific nerves to block the body's messages of pain heading to the brain. It works for many types and areas of pain from many different causes.

Some believe that the same stabs of electrical energy also cause the body to release endorphins. Endorphins are natural pain relievers that the body makes.

The TENS equipment comes complete with a belt battery pack, the stimulator, and wires from it to the electrodes held onto the skin by a patch. The electrodes are placed on the painful muscles and can be stimulated by the electrical charge automatically on a continuous basis, or set so the patient can turn the charge on and off to use just when needed.

TENS has been around for years, and can be effective, depending on the individual. Talk to your doctor to see if it would work for you.

MAGNETISM

Sometimes the pain is so bad that a patient will try almost anything for relief. Many FMS people have reported good relief with the use of good old, everyday magnets. This kind of simple, inexpensive and drugless therapy comes in waves of popularity. Now and then you'll see a major sports star who says that he or she uses magnets all the time for pain relief.

The idea is that the magnetic field stimulates or interacts with the normal electrical system of the body. The theory is that this can increase blood circulation, decrease pain and reduce inflammation.

Some believe that a magnet on a sore muscle will interfere with the pain signals getting through to the brain. They also think that the magnets stimulate the body's natural painkillers, the endorphins.

Who can say if magnets work or not? There have been few scientific studies in this area. One was done at Baylor University and another is underway, paid for by the National Institutes of Health at the University of Virginia. There probably is a placebo effect of 15 to 20 percent, from the psychological benefits, that makes so many people think the magnet works, so they actually do have a reduction in pain.

Side effects? Some people have complained of headaches, insomnia and backache after extended periods of magnet use.

But it's not clear if the magnets or something else caused these problems. For now, you pays your money and you takes your chances. If nothing else works for you, you might want to give the magnets a chance.

INJECTIONS

Injections of local anesthetics with a small dose of a cortisone derivative have been used for many years in all sorts of situations and for all types of pain. They will work as well on your FMS pains.

They will give temporary relief especially at painful trigger points. It may take a few days for the relief to come, but when it does it can last for weeks. This treatment is especially good if you are getting better in many areas from your FMS, but one or two painful muscles remain. The local injections can clear up the last of the tough pain.

Side effects? Usually there are none and no problems. The cortisone does not affect the rest of the body.

Injections of the same type can also be done around the spine for epidural, facet joints and nerve blocks. These injections can sometimes give relief from pain, and last for several months. The injections can be repeated without any harmful effects.

ULTRASOUND

These high frequency sound waves can be used on the muscles and tendons of the soft tissue on the back and shoulders. Often used with deep heat, ultrasound can help in relaxation, improve pain in tender points and even decrease inflammation. Usually this is done by a physical therapist over a series of treatments. It can be continued if it gives relief without any side effects.

DRINK, FOOD AND DRUG INTERACTION

Be careful to follow closely the directions and cautions that you receive with every medication you buy at your pharmacy. This is especially important if you drink alcohol.

Most medications tell you whether to take them on an

empty stomach or with food. Some say eat half your meal, take the medication, then eat the rest of the food. Follow this instruction.

If a medication says don't take with alcohol, or to drink water after taking the medication, obey that directive. Ignoring it can result in serious trouble—and even death.

If you drink alcohol with an anti-depressant, your intoxication can be extreme and dangerous. If you have a muscle relaxant and drink alcohol, your brain activity will be seriously depressed. By drinking alcohol when taking sleeping pills, you can cause serious over-sedation that can result in your death.

Follow the rules, stay healthier and stay alive.

COMBINING MEDICATION WITH TREATMENTS

When it comes to deep muscle pain, many doctors suggest you fight it this way:

- wet heat: shower, tub, pool
- exercise: pick the best one for you
- an anti-depressant medication
- a nonsterodial anti-inflammatory drug.

You will find that it might take some experimentation to come up with the right drugs that work the best for you. It's worth it. Once you tie down the right combination, you should have a good run at dragging down your pain to a practical, workable level that will allow you much more normal activity.

TIPS FOR USING YOUR MEDICATIONS

If your symptoms don't lessen, or even increase, you may need a larger dose to make it work. Ask your doctor.

Sometimes a small dose of a medication is needed. Pill cutters are available to slice pills neatly in half.

Some people only need medication during symptom flare-ups—ask your doctor for a plan for flare-ups. This might mean starting or increasing a medication. It might be needed for four or five nights. A second medication might also be needed.

It might help to take part of your nighttime medicine in the evening and the rest at bedtime. It might help you sleep better and avoid that hangover feeling when awakening.

If you take part of your evening medication in the daytime, it could help loosen muscles and relieve pain.

Remember, some antidepressants can alleviate depression, but may not help you get the deep sleep that you need.

Be prepared for a flare-up. Ask your doctor how much you can increase your medication when a serious flare-up comes. Get guidelines. That way you won't have to try to get in touch to get permission to increase your medication.

This same "increase instruction" should be used for bouts of sleeplessness, and premenstrually. Some people increase medications during winter months or in hot and humid months when symptoms become more aggravated.

CHAPTER 4

OTHER MEDICAL TREATMENTS

Many people with FMS keep a journal or a diary of their aches and pains and treatments and medications. This is a great idea. If you don't want to go that far, it is still a fine plan to keep a record of what medications you are taking. Put down the date you started, the name of the medication, the dosage, the doctor's name, and then a column showing the response, side effects, increases or decreases in dosage and what the end result was.

Most FMS patients go through a litany of types of drugs. It is beneficial to you and your doctor for you to be able to show at a glance what medications you have had and what worked and what didn't. The doctor could dig it out of your medical file, but by now it's over three inches thick and she might not have that much time.

A spiral bound 8.5 x 11-inch school pad makes a good place for your chart. It's cheap, easy to store, and to take with you when you go see your doctor.

MULTIPLE DRUG THERAPY?

Almost always, one medication is not enough to treat the several symptoms of those with FMS. For example, one drug might be used to relieve the pain, but another would be needed to handle the muscle tightness situation. Later, another medication would be prescribed to handle the sleep problem.

Combining drugs usually means that smaller doses of each can be used. So far the combination of drugs works as well as single drugs, but researchers hope in the future that drugs working together will work much better than singly.

CONSULT A PSYCHIATRIST

Yes, in some cases it works well to consult with a psychiatrist before prescribing medications for those with anxiety and depression. Most psychiatrists have a great deal of experience with these two problems and have prescribed hundreds of times. They know which drugs work the best.

This works only when a doctor refers the patient when he knows the patient has FMS. If the doctor doesn't know what the patient has, usually the psychiatrist won't discover it either, and the patient is the one who suffers.

DEPRESSION MEDICATIONS

There may be a chemical imbalance in the brain that causes depression and other fibromyalgia problems. Depression might also arise from the frustration of fatigue and sleeplessness and chronic pain and other symptoms of FMS.

Prescriptions to treat sleep disturbances and pain are often lower in strength than those needed to treat depression. However, these doses can sometimes work to reduce an FMS depression. For some patients a three-month prescription for anti-depressant drugs can alter an underlying chemical imbalance and dramatically reduce or eliminate the depression. If depression is not treated in an FMS patient, it will adversely affect other symptoms and the patient's lifestyle.

TENDER POINT INJECTIONS?

Tender points, those eighteen spots on the body that show a marked painful response when pressured, might be helped with injections of anesthetic and/or cortisone. The only problem is, most of the tender points hurt when palpated. Few FMS patients would want to have eighteen injections, and the cost would be prohibitive.

WILL ACUPUNCTURE HELP?

Patients strongly in favor of acupuncture usually are not discouraged. Some of the eighteen tender points correspond to the acupuncture points. Usually patients with FMS do not benefit from acupuncture, except for related emotional and psychosomatic help. If other treatments have not helped a patient, acupuncture is worth a try. Most doctors can refer you to a qualified person. Some physicians and neurologists now offer acupuncture.

PHYSICAL THERAPY

If your physical therapist understands what fibromyalgia is and what it does to your body, he or she may be able to help you.

Treatments designed for loosening tight muscles, relieving pain, stretching and conditioning muscles, and preventing such problems, can be given by a PT with good results.

If you have flare-ups, your doctor may order a heat treatment to counter intense pain. The heat treatment can be followed by deep massage to relieve muscle tightness and spasms. This heat and massage can shorten the flare-up.

As a substitute for a professional heat treatment, try a hot shower or bath for from fifteen to thirty minutes, twice a day, for a week. It just might help.

OCCUPATIONAL THERAPY

Bad posture and poor work-related positions won't cause fibromyalgia, but, over time, they can cause strains and aggravate FMS related pains. An occupational therapist can check your work related positions and your posture and perhaps make suggestions that will help keep you from making worse any FMS pains. For example you might have neck and shoulder FMS pains. How you sit at your computer might be making those pains much worse. Your OT can make suggestions to improve your work positions to help prevent them from making your FMS pains worse.

BIOFEEDBACK CAN HELP

Yes, biofeedback can make a difference in your FMS pains. The experts say that biofeedback can increase blood levels of endorphins and hormones in your body.

The purpose of biofeedback here is to regulate posture and structural movement, and release muscle tension to reduce pain.

Computers linked to sensors on the body provide video and audio readouts of your reactions. The therapist helps the patient to relax muscles while he or she can see the results on the readout.

Breathing often becomes shallow and irregular when a person has pains. Lower breath rate lowers the delivery of oxygen to muscles. Biofeedback shows the patient how to breathe deep and regularly and then exhale fully, which helps relax tension.

THERAPEUTIC MASSAGE

We've mentioned massage before. This is the full course. Massage can loosen tight muscles, promote deep muscle relaxation, increase circulation, reduce stress, and relieve pain and spasms. A trained physical therapist will use heat in association with massage to relax tight and painful muscles.

Tell your PT that you have fibromyalgia. If the therapist doesn't know what that is, explain it, and what you want to have done. Show the therapist where you hurt the most. You'll have to tell the PT if the massage is too strong or too light. Make sure that the therapist understands that the massage is only a part of your overall program and not a cure in itself.

MEDITATION AND RELAXATION

Some FMS people say that meditation and relaxation training

has been helpful in reducing pain and fatigue. This takes a special instructor, or there are some audiotapes that do the same thing. The idea is to learn to relax your muscles for twenty minutes each day. This is a part of the idea that the more you can do yourself to help resolve your FMS, the better.

MASSAGE

Massage may help your muscle pain. Muscles can build up lactic acid. Massage, in its various forms, may help disperse this acid and relieve the pain. Proponents say that massage can also heighten alertness, lower the level of stress hormones, cut down on sleep problems and help relieve depression and anxiety.

Some FMS patients report that after a massage they needed fewer drugs to combat muscle pain, and that their heart rate decreased and their blood pressure went down.

One type of massage works on the trigger points. This is said to help relieve muscle spasms and cramping. The active trigger points are located, and mild to moderate pressure is exerted for seven to ten seconds. The muscles are then stretched gently to help in relaxation.

ACUPRESSURE

This type of physical therapy predates acupuncture, and uses many of the same pressure points that acupuncture does. It works by stimulating your body's main trigger points. This is done to release energy and to unblock *qi*—the life force. Acupressure may not be effective on FMS patients. It is mostly used to work on other ailments such as sinus pressure, leg cramps and headaches.

QIGONG

This form of Chinese medicine is reported to increase energy, alleviate pain and decrease fatigue. All of these sound good to an FMS patient. This is one of the first of the Chinese healing techniques. When doing this, you will move into specific physical postures to help ease tension over your whole body.

This is a technique you'll have to learn. It may require you to pay a practitioner to teach you how to do it. Sometimes classes are available at a community center. After you know the positions and movements, you can do these by yourself. Those who use this program say they need less medication and heal faster. The secret is to do the postures and exercises every morning.

CHIROPRACTIC

This is a drug-free approach to health, and uses manipulation of the muscles and the spine to cure your ills. Does it work? It depends who you talk to.

Chiropractors deal mainly with your spinal column. They say it is the seat of all problems, since all signals from the brain go down the spinal column to the various muscles and tendons. Pain signals go back the other way. By adjusting and correcting the position of the vertebrae in the spine, they say they can solve many of your problems.

HYDROTHERAPY

We talked about the advantages of a hot shower, tub bath, whirlpool or even a heated pool. The heat relaxes the muscles and brings a bit of immediate relief from aching and painful muscles.

Cold compresses will also help. The practice is to use cold on a new problem such as a sprained ankle, injured hand or arm, pulled muscle or anywhere that there is swelling. The cold helps reduce the swelling, and in some cases running cold water over a wound will help reduce any swelling and rid it of bacteria.

Icing a hurt is seen at sports events, especially at college and pro football games. Ice and heat are easily obtainable. Use them for injuries, and to see if they will cut down on your deep muscle pain.

HYPNOTHERAPY

Yes, hypnosis can have a beneficial effect on your FMS symptoms. It is a good way to help control pain and stress and is recommended by the American Psychiatric Association.

In some cases, those who use hypnotherapy say they have better results in controlling pain, fatigue and poor sleep patterns than they have had under physical therapy.

The post-hypnotic suggestion routine has been used to help patients ease muscle pain, even to move the pain from one area to another where it is less pronounced.

One of the best times to try hypnotherapy is when nothing else is working, or high doses of drugs are needed to get the desired relief from deep pain, depression and stress. As you may have seen in demonstrations, hypnosis is not right for every patient. In fact some people can't be hypnotized because they simply refuse to be.

If the idea appeals to you, first see a qualified psychologist or psychiatrist to see if he or she recommends that you try the hypnosis track to help relieve your pains.

LAUGHTER THERAPY

Don't laugh at this idea. Well, go ahead, it could help. Many researchers today say that laughter increases the activity of cells that attack viruses and tumor cells. It also helps to relieve anxiety, increases the immune system action, and decreases stress-producing hormones.

Scientists today say that laugher alone can produce a positive state in the body they call eustress. In a California test, researchers found that laugher alone produced significant increases in the immune system, especially T cells and KK cells. Also the stress hormone cortisol, which suppresses the immune system, was shown to be lower after the laughter experiment.

So, why not have a good laugh—get out those old funny movies or rent some good video yuckers. It just might help and it can't hurt. Go ahead, laugh.

CHAPTER 5

IS GUAIFENESIN THE MAGICAL CURE?

Dr. R. Paul St. Amand, M.D., endocrinologist and UCLA assistant clinical professor, says that almost anyone who uses the drug guaifenesin the proper way can reverse the pains and agonies of fibromyalgia.

He bases his statement on forty years of research into the aches and pains and fatigue and ailments that were eventually called fibromyalgia, and his experiences with hundreds of patients with the syndrome.

He says that the use of guaifenesin—an inexpensive, long-used ingredient in most cough syrups—can reverse and in some cases eliminate entirely the problems caused by fibromyalgia in 90 percent of the victims.

WHAT IS GUAIFENESIN?

Guaifenesin is one of the ingredients in most cough syrups, used for loosening phlegm in the throat. In liquid form, it is also an active ingredient in many expectorants and sinus preparations. It is a tree bark extract, and first noted in 1530 when it was used for rheumatism and later for gout. In 1928 it was used for what was called "growing pains" and some other symptoms that today we call fibromyalgia. It was first used in cough mixtures more than seventy years ago.

The patent on it has long since lapsed, and it is made by several firms and is available over-the-counter in 600 mg tablets at a cost of around $30 for 100 pills. The drug has no side effects.

HOW DOES IT WORK ON FIBROMYALGIA?

Dr. St. Amand says that he believes that the cause of fibromyalgia is a defective kidney that works well except that it is short one basic necessary ability. It simply can't expel all of the accumulated wastes in the bloodstream. He believes that the problem here is inorganic phosphate. Usually there is a control in the kidney that can in effect open a faucet and let out the excess waste products. Those with fibromyalgia don't have this "open faucet" to get rid of the products.

The blood brings the normal amount of inorganic phosphates to the kidneys and they simply can't eliminate all of it, so much of the waste is recirculated in the blood. He says that a defective enzyme is responsible for this problem. As our cells produce energy they produce a great many inorganic phosphates in normal functioning. Those with fibromyalgia can't expel enough of it, and some of the phosphates are absorbed into the body tissues because they have no place else to go. This absorption is what causes the muscle pain, Dr. St. Amand says.

So, how does guaifenesin help? The theory is that guaifenesin helps the enzymes in the kidneys to open those spigots and pump out the offending inorganic phosphates that are doing all of the damage in the bones and fibers of the body.

These excesses of phosphates also interrupt the regular production of energy by the body. That further hurts the person with fibromyalgia and results in fatigue, sleeplessness and the other symptoms.

With the use of guaifenesin, the patient will at first have worse symptoms than he or she had before. As this process of reversal begins, the phosphates must be drained out of the fibers and bones of the body. This simply makes the hurt worse in all aspects.

With a low dose of guaifenesin, 300 mg two times a day, a

patient will experience attacks of the FMS symptoms for two to three weeks. After that the patient will start to feel better in groups of hours, then in a day here and there and, when all of the reversal is over, all or most of the symptoms will be gone.

This medication can't reverse damage done to the body by fibromyalgia or by any medications, but it can reverse and eliminate most of the fibromyalgia symptoms, Dr. St. Amand says.

SALICYLATES CAN BLOCK GUAIFENESIN

The bad guys here are the many and various forms of salicylate—the best known is the common aspirin. Today salicylates can be made synthetically. They also exist in almost all plants and help the plants to counteract bacteria in the soil. Without the plant's natural salicylate, it could never grow out of the ground.

Salicylates have been used by man for as far back as the fifth century B.C. when Hippocrates used a juice extracted from the bark of willow trees to treat his patients' aches and pains.

It was first synthesized in Germany in 1893 as acetylsalicylic acid, and was called aspirin.

For anyone being treated with guaifenesin, aspirin and all salicylates are the deadliest of enemies. That's because salicylates absolutely block any benefits that guaifenesin could give.

In short that means cutting out everything in your diet and your life that involves salicylates—and that means roughly about half the products you use. Salicylates can easily be absorbed through the skin and are found in many cosmetics.

What products contain salicylates? Some include:

- Aspirin
- Ginkgo-biloba
- Dong Kwai
- Preparation H
- St. John's Wort
- Vicks Cough drops
- Aloe Vera Gel
- Milk of Magnesia

- Vicks Vaporub Cream
- Alka Seltzer
- Anacin
- Ben Gay
- Bufferin
- Pepto Bismol
- Clearasil
- Coppertone Sunblock
- Listerex Scrub Lotion
- Noxema
- Stridex Scrub pads

That's just a sample. Thousands of items, many that are used by most people every day, contain salicylates. Cosmetics are included.

If you take guaifenesin you must read every label to see if the product contains any salicylates. Rigorously throw away all that do, and don't buy any more. It can be a monumental problem.

How to Use Guaifenesin

Find a doctor who understands fibromyalgia, knows that it is a treatable disease, and will help you. This can be a GP or an internist. You don't need a specialist.

Find a doctor who also will put you on the guaifenesin program and keep you on it with checks along the way. This might not be so easy to find, since guaifenesin may be an untried and unproven treatment for many.

Once you have a doctor who knows you have fibromyalgia and has tested you for other similar ailments and has ruled them out, have your body "mapped" for bumps and lumps from the fibromyalgia. This should also include hardened muscle areas. If your doctor or nurse won't do this, have them suggest a physical therapist they trust to do the job. This will give you a base line to check as your treatment goes along.

Now, eliminate all salicylates from your life.

This one is tougher. You'll need to clean out your medicine cabinet and check labels to see what has salicylates in it. Simply throw them all out. Get replacement products for the same job without the salicylates.

Do the same for your cosmetic kit and shelf. It might kill you, but get rid of any cosmetic, even your favorite lipstick, that has salicylates in it.

Do the same thing for your refrigerator, food shelf, pantry, wherever you store your food. Read the labels. You'll be surprised what has salicylates in it.

If you're a gardener, and work with the soil, always wear sturdy, waterproof gloves. The soil itself can give you enough skin-absorbed salicylates to completely block and negate your guaifenesin regimen.

Get a prescription from your doctor for guaifenesin. It will have an "LA" on it somewhere standing for Long Acting. Make sure the pills you get contain only guaifenesin and nothing else. There will be a number, usually 600 mg or 1200 mg. If the numbers are 600/150, it may indicate two medications. Check with the pharmacist.

This drug works for twelve hours, so take it twice a day, when you get up in the morning, then about twelve hours later.

Most patients begin with 300 mg twice a day. If you don't feel worse during the first week, talk to your doctor about increasing the dosage to 600 mg twice a day. Yes, you should feel *WORSE*, not better, after a week or two. Remember, you're reversing the damage.

You and your doctor decide when you should be mapped again. The mapping will show improvement when it comes. After the first month you should begin to have some of those good hours, and then good days that soon should blend into a good week.

With guaifenesin there is that period of reversal where you will feel much worse than usual, but this period will be followed by your feeling better.

If this is not happening with you, ask your doctor to increase your dosage. This is not dangerous, because guaifenesin has no side effects. Some patients may need 1800 mg a day, or up to 3600 mg. If this isn't working, check closely your salicylate intake. You must be having a blockage of the drug. Look again at your labels. If you've kept that favorite lipstick or wrinkle cream that you know has salicylate, pitch it out.

How long do you take the medication? As long as you need it to reverse fibromyalgia and to get rid of all or most of the pains and exhaustion and sleeplessness. You will have a therapeutic level that you need to keep fibromyalgia away. If you go below that, the pains may come back.

DOES IT WORK?

Dr. St. Amand says he has hundred of patients to prove that it does work. He has a book out on the subject: *What Your Doctor May Not Tell You About Fibromyalgia*. It is by Dr. R. Paul St. Amand and Claudia Craig Marek. It's a paperback published by Warner Books, sells for $14.95 and if your bookstore doesn't have it, they can order it for you.

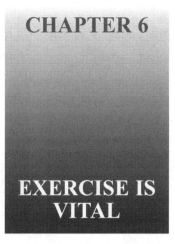

CHAPTER 6

EXERCISE IS VITAL

You say your muscles hurt and you don't want to even take a walk? Exercise is the last thing you want to hear about, let alone do?

Mistake. Wrong. No way, Jose. Not a chance. Give it up.

Experts on FMS now say that the correct type of exercise program is one of the best medications you can take to recover and maintain good health. True. Even five years ago, exercise was not thought to be good for aching muscles.

Now the reverse is true. Why? Regular exercise activates your whole body, gets more blood circulating and is generally good for whole body health. Exercise helps prevent other problems not associated with FMS such as heart disease, diabetes, obesity and high blood pressure.

You say your legs hurt, so how can you take a half-mile walk?

Give it a try. Believing you can take that walk is half the battle.

How does exercise help your FMS? It promotes blood circulation—getting blood to nourish your bodily tissues. Exercise increases your flexibility, helps produce more healing endorphins in your immune system, helps promote the secretion of serotonin and growth hormones, and increases the production of T-cells in your autoimmune system.

Exercise of the right kind and in the right amount is also important in weight control, increasing mobility and reducing pain. It also helps your joints and supportive structures such as ligaments and tendons—vital for FMS patients.

Fibromyalgia victims, who stop all kinds of exercise, even walking around the house, soon find out that they have made a mistake. When muscles are not used, they tend to shrink and weaken. The lack of exercise will further increase the pain and other problems from FMS. It's a cycle that soon deteriorates the body—which makes the FMS symptoms worse than before.

Activity and planned exercises have exactly the opposite effect on the body and on FMS symptoms.

Let's take a look at how exercise fights the painful effects of fibromyalgia:

- Exercise helps strengthen tendons and ligaments, and promotes muscle tone.
- When your body is well-toned, and has strong muscles, tendons and ligaments, they will do their regular work of supporting the body, and help lessen pain.
- Blood flow to muscles increases with exercise.
- More blood flowing to your muscles means more oxygen and nutrients get to the muscles and fibers. This helps to restore depleted muscles and re-supplies the muscle tissue. Most FMS patients have a lower blood flow than normal. Anything we can do to increase that—such as exercise—will help reduce pain.
- The growth of T-cells is helped by exercise.
- After exercise, the thymus gland produces a larger number of the killer T-cells than it does normally. This is vitally important to the FMS person. T-cells enhance the autoimmune system. The T-cells are the body's fighters, attacking most disease cells. Both of these increases help the body work itself back toward normal.

EXERCISE HELPS FLEXIBILITY AND RANGE
OF MOTION

Flexible and pliable muscles simply work better and will help you to avoid muscle tears, strains or pulls. Exercise helps your muscles be more flexible. The more flexible your muscle are, the easier it is to do normal actions such as walking, stooping, reaching, and even sitting.

Exercise can prevent muscle stiffness, which is one of the early morning problems for FMS patients. You can probably reduce or eliminate that morning stiffness with exercise. The more and better you exercise, the better your whole body will function—including overall muscle and joint working. This can result in less pain and less tension—which can work on lowering your stress.

ENDORPHIN PRODUCTION INCREASES

Endorphins in your body help with healing, are a natural pain reliever, and help you to get better deep sleep. When you exercise, the action increases the production of endorphins and their release into your body to help you feel better.

OLD FRIEND SEROTONIN

Yes, it's back. Serotonin production is increased with exercise. You've heard this before. Remember it this time. Serotonin and its growth hormone enhancement are two of the agents that most FMS patients lack. They are pain reducers and muscle-repair materials that can help you to feel better.

SYNOVIAL FLUID...A HOUSEHOLD TERM

Synovial fluid moves in and out of your joints as they function. With exercise, the joints work more, and more of this fluid washes out of the cartilage, lubricates it and brings in nourishment to keep the joints healthy—and so they will hurt a lot less for an FMS patient.

Now, a little review about what exercise can do to help a person with fibromyalgia. Remember these, then get to exercising.

PROMOTES RELAXATION. Helps ward off anxiety and depression. Decreases insulin resistance and aids the control of your blood sugar level. Aids in the treatment of diabetes. Lowers blood fats and increases the good cholesterol. This helps to cut down on your chance of coronary heart disease or a stroke.

RELAXES TENSION AND MAY INCREASE YOUR DEEP SLEEP LEVEL TO LEVEL FOUR. Tones and strengthens the organs and systems in your body. Helps you increase self-control and mental efficiency. Also will help your feeling of well being and your own emotional power.

WILL IMPROVE YOUR ELIMINATION PROCESS AND RELIEVE CONSTIPATION. Lengthens your life span. Will aid in protecting you against osteoporosis and arthritis. Improves your body by lowering body fat percentage and building up your muscles. Increases your endurance and strength for both play and work.

THERE ARE THREE DEFINITIONS OF PHYSICAL FITNESS

They are *muscular strength*, *muscle flexibility* and *cardiovascular fitness*.

We'll look at these individually in a moment—first a word about you and an exercise program. You've probably heard that no one should start an exercise or cardiovascular program without first getting a good physical examination and then talking it over with your doctor.

This applies doubly for persons with FMS. It just makes sense.

After your exam, your doctor can either suggest which exercises you should not do, or help you work out a fitness program. Some physicians may refer you to a physical therapist to devise an exercise program for you that will not aggravate any of your FMS symptoms and still do the job.

Okay, on with the program:

MUSCULAR STRENGTH

At one time the strength exercises were all anyone did. The

"pumping iron" syndrome had been firmly established. The idea that strong muscles can get those hundreds of daily living tasks done better than weak ones is still true. It's like a big luxury car with a 300 horsepower engine steaming up a hill at 50 miles an hour. It's using about a fifth of its total power. Behind it is a small car with a hundred horsepower grinding up the same hill at 50 miles an hour. The difference is the small car is using about 80% of its power. The conclusion is that the big car's engine will last a lot longer than the small car's since it's not working nearly as hard as the small car engine.

Same for our bodies. Strong muscles do the same job much easier than weak ones. Strength training? You can do it by lifting free weights in a gym or in your living room, by working out on weight machines in a gym, or using a resistance device as simple as an elastic tube. These are great for a number of different exercises including simple curls.

Don't think you have to bench press 400 pounds to get into shape. You might start with five or ten pounds on your curls, or light resistance on the various machines. The idea is to get into a program and stay with it, building up on your weights as you can as the weight gets easier. A physical therapist can help you here.

Yes, you can hurt yourself with free weights if you don't know what you're doing. If you workout at a gym, get instruction what to do and how to do it. Follow the regimen. You'll want to get used to the weights, you'll want to progress to heavier ones. How often to work out with the weights? If you work out at home, make it six days a week. At a gym probably three or four times a week.

The important point is to establish a program you can continue and then work it religiously. You'll notice a difference.

MUSCULAR FLEXIBILITY

Have you ever watched a ballet dancer warming up? Fascinating. These dancer/athletes specialize in flexibility. They are remarkable, doing splits flat on the floor, kicking high over their heads and bending in ways that constantly amaze.

They work at flexibility so they can do the movements required.

Flexibility is just as important to everyone, especially those with FMS. You'll never do what the ballet dancer can do, but the more flexing you can get the better. If you try to do something as simple as bending over and your muscles are too tight and stiff from not doing any exercising for a long time, that bending over could create too much stress on your muscles and you could injure yourself.

Simple stretching movements that your physical therapist can show you can do wonders for your other forms of exercise. What are some of them? Yoga in its non-meditation form, some of the martial arts, and the use of the stretching elastic tube which can be used in literally dozens of different ways for stretching and strength.

CARDIOVASCULAR FITNESS

You know this term. It simply means how well your heart and lungs can furnish the blood, oxygen and nutrients your body needs for physical activity. Another way of saying it is aerobic capacity.

Exercises that build up your cardiovascular system also help to strengthen your joints and work on your bone health as well.

What exercises are good for increasing your aerobic capacity?

Aerobic dancing. True, but most of these are designed for overactive young adults and are not good for those with FMS. They simply go too fast, too hard and too long.

Let's start out with something easier like stationary bike riding, walking, biking, jogging, stair climbing, swimming, rowing, even western line dancing and square dancing can apply.

The rule here is that the workout must be continuous and keep your pulse going for twenty to twenty-five minutes. This length of time lets your body have a good workout and works your heart and lungs and circulation system.

Here you'll want to talk to your doctor or Physical Therapist for help in choosing what kind of aerobic exercise you should do, and for how long. The extent of your fibromyalgia may limit what you can do. Always work up to the maximum you can, depending on your physical condition.

Don't be upset if you need to start out slow, even on a treadmill for ten or fifteen minutes at a time, or on a stationary bike for about the same time. Now you can have the enjoyment of watching your development as you get stronger.

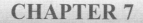

CHAPTER 7

LET'S START YOUR EXERCISE PROGRAM

Before You Charge Forth: Your first job in setting up your exercise program is to check out the idea with your regular doctor. She knows you and your condition. Ask her if there are any exercises or programs that you should not do. Then if she agrees that you can start an exercise workout program, ask her what you should do. She may refer you to a Physical Therapist for a set of exercises or the type of workout that will help you and your fibromyalgia the most.

Working on your cardiovascular system and stretching and strengthening muscles can be done safely and with good effect for almost every FMS patient. That includes you.

If you have a flare-up of pain or other symptom of your FMS, ask your doctor what you should do. She might tell you to avoid the more physical exercises and limit yourself to slow walking or riding a stationary bike for a day or two until the flare-up eases down. If the pains continue, you may need to take a break from your exercise program until your flare-up is over.

Remember that physical exercise is a vital part of any treatment program for FMS. Even a simple aerobic exercise plan can help avoid muscle atrophy and will help with other aspects of your condition.

If you haven't been active lately, start a physical fitness program gradually. Warm up before any workout. This might be a five-minute stretching routine. Then to get off to a start, you might do five or ten minutes of walking. Whatever workout you pick, be sure it's something you enjoy doing. If you don't enjoy it, you won't last long at it. Be sure the program is convenient. If you have to drive twenty miles to get to the gym or pool or walking area, it won't be long before you find reasons not to go.

Walking is a fine exercise, it's always close by, and you don't need a partner or team or pool or court to do it.

Some common sense rules for your exercise:

AVOID TOO MUCH TOO SOON. Too much can lead to an injury or strain that will stop your program. It's good to try to do a little more than you did last week. After a week's activity at one level—say walking a quarter mile—is a good time slot to move up your distance or reps. Don't push yourself too hard. Learn the difference between a small increase, and an over-zealous drive to injury.

LISTEN TO YOUR BODY. Know and recognize the signals that your body is sending you. You might feel great, or you might get dizzy, feel chest pain, get nauseous, or get short of breath. If any of these happen, stop your exercise and rest. Decide if the exercise is at fault, or if the pains are a one-time thing.

BEGIN YOUR PROGRAM SLOWLY. Start out at a reasonable level for your age and condition. Don't compete with anyone. Feel comfortable in your workout. Build your times or reps gradually and your body will strengthen as you go.

SORE MUSCLE OR A TEAR? You probably will be a little muscle stiff and sore the first few days. Learn to recognize this stiffness from what could be a muscle strain or tear. If the hurt goes away quickly as you stretch, it's just stiffness.

ALWAYS WARM-UP. This is a must for any physical activity except walking, which is a form of warm-up for more strenuous workouts. Warming up will help increase blood flow, warm those muscles you'll be using and increase your body heat. A good warm-up will make a better workout.

ALWAYS COOL DOWN. This is a gradual slowing of your heart rate and your temperature to get your body back to normal. Depending how strenuous your workout is, pick something to let you slow down gradually. If you bicycle or swim, a good cool out is to walk a quarter of a mile or so. You'll slow down your system. Cooling out properly will help reduce any muscle soreness and eliminate the lactic acid from your muscles.

THE EXERCISES

WALKING

Walking is the easiest form of exercise there is. You can do it in a mall, right outside your door and around the block. You don't need a partner to play with or against. You can set your own pace, and go for any distance that you want to. Nobody will yell at you to play through or go faster or get out of the way.

Walking is a complete exercise, working your legs, but also your arms if you swing them or bounce a ball. Walking is effective and enjoyable and will help you to lose weight and maintain or restore your health.

How? Walking burns fat and calories, boosts your energy level, strengthens and tones your muscles, improves muscle flexibility, eliminates muscle pain and improves energy production. You realize that all of these things help the person with fibromyalgia.

Which is better, to walk fast for a short distance, or to walk a little slower for a longer distance? Pick the longer distance and you'll be a winner. It also gives your aerobic system more of a workout and that's good.

As with any new exercise, you should start out slowly. At first walk for from ten to twenty minutes. Plan a circular trip around your neighborhood so you can get back to your rocking chair by the time your designated time is over. If you walk north for twenty minutes, it figures that you'll have to do twenty minutes of walking south to get back to where you started.

Do your minimum walk for a week. It's best to do it every day, or at least six times a week. The second week bump it up five minutes, and go for a week that way. Increase it weekly until you get to your ideal target time of about 45 minutes. This time gives your heart and lungs a good aerobic workout as well as your legs and arms.

HEART RATE

For any exercise, you should try to keep your heart beating at the ideal number of throbs. You find out this magic number by first learning to take your own pulse. The carotid artery in both sides of your neck is the easiest place to find your pulse. Count it for a minute when you are resting. Write it down.

Now write down the figure 220, then subtract your age, say 45. That leaves 175. Now subtract that resting heart beat that you just counted out. Say it was 65. Now you have 110. Then multiply that number by .65 and that gives you 72. Now add your resting heart rate, 65, to the 72 and you have 137. This is your maximum heart beat rate.

For best aerobic results you should exercise with your heartbeat at about 70 percent of that maximum, or in this case 70 percent of 137 is 96. So try to keep your heart beat around 100 when you're exercising.

The easy way to do this is to count your heartbeats for ten seconds and multiply by six. Say your beat for ten seconds is 16. You multiply that times six and you get 96, your exact projected 70 percent of your maximum.

If your heart beat is twenty after a mile run, that works out to 120 beats which is way over your ideal. So next time run slower or don't go up those steep hills.

Back to walking. If you can keep your heart beat at about 70 percent while you're walking, you can maintain that workout for a long period of time and give your muscles and heart and lungs a good session and perhaps also lose weight.

Can a walking program cause you to lose weight? It will on

most people. Your own metabolic system may be different. But give it a try. Look at it this way. If you walk thirty minutes a day, that should cover about two miles. Six days a week gives you 12 miles a week or 48 miles a month. At this distance you'll be burning up about 1500 calories a week. If you burn up 3500 calories, you will burn away one pound of weight. So with 1500 calories times four weeks, gives you 9,000 calories a month. That means you are dropping almost three pounds a month. A good moderate weight loss. If you boost your walking to four miles a day you will double your weight loss to six pounds a month, one and a half a week.

THE OLD FOOTPADS

A good pair of walking shoes is important. That doesn't mean expensive. There are sturdy, well cushioned shoes on the market for $20. You don't have to pay $65 or $120 to get practical walking shoes. If you buy a name brand you're paying way too much. At least half your cost is for the brand name.

THE PSYCHOLOGICAL PART

Positive thinking will help your exercise program. When working to restore your health, food is important and the exercises, too, so now let's throw in positive thinking. You know this is going to work. You understand how exercise, like walking, helps to rejuvenate the body, and it will help lower your problems with FMS. Such positive thinking helps your self-esteem and even helps raise your metabolic rate.

WALK EVERY DAY

What? No time off? Okay, take Sunday off, but the other six days are a must. Get it down in your exercise diary how long you walked and how far. This will be a valuable record as the days and weeks pass. You can look back and see how far you've come—and how far you've traveled—in such a little time. Make your walking a definite part of your daily routine. Would it work best before you go to work, before the day really begins, or is it better in the late afternoon or evening? Work it out. Then do the work.

WALK SIX DAYS A WEEK

Yes, we just said that, so this is for emphasis. You are working to restore your good health, to kick FMS right in the old chops and get back to better things. Takes work. Takes commitment. One of those things is to do your exercises six days a week. Build your walking routine into your daily schedule. Make it so you'll not feel quite right if you don't do your walk. After your day's break of not walking, you should be eager to get back to it on the next day. Give it a try. Actually you have nothing to lose by giving it a six-month try.

THE TIME AND THE DISTANCE

You put in the time, you'll get the distance. As we said before, you won't get there in a day. Start slow and work up. You'll be surprised how quickly you'll be moving from twenty to thirty minutes of walking. Try to average a mile every fifteen minutes. It's not a fast pace, but you can't stop to pat the dogs along the way, either. The longer you walk, the more calories you'll burn off and the better your aerobic workout will be. Your heart and your lungs will thank you.

THE OLD WARM UP

You don't need to do much stretching for your warm up for walking. About the best one is to try to push a tree over. Lean forward at about a 45-degree angle and feel your Achilles tendon stretch. Let your knees lower a little and you'll feel the tendons back there working. You may want to do some other minor stretching but it's not really needed for walking. In fact, walking is used as a warm up for other exercises. You may want to start out at a slower walk and then speed it up when you feel like your muscles are warm and your blood is pumping. This might take a quarter of a mile or so.

CLOTHING AND SHOES

We talked about shoes before. Repetition is a good educational process. Some runners will not wear a pair of expensive running shoes for more than 500 miles. They say they are broken down by then. For them 500 miles might only be five weeks of intensive training before a marathon. Any good pair of running or walking shoes will do. And remember that $20 pair of shoes. They are around. The rest of your clothes should be loose fitting and comfortable. Light shorts and T-shirt in summer, a pair of sweats and cap in the winter. Yeah, walk every day, rain, shine or snow.

WHERE TO WALK

At first, stick to flat sidewalks around your neighborhood, especially if there are no steep hills. This gives you a good way to get in your miles and stay close to home. As your distance lengthens, you may try a park, hiking trails, high school track or athletic field, or, for more advanced walking, pick out a series of good-sized hills and trek up and down them. That will put an added burden on your legs, heart and lungs. Work up to the hills.

BICYCLING

The second most popular form of exercise for many fibromyalgia patients is bicycling. Many of the same benefits apply. There is little in equipment needed: just a bike and a helmet. You can use any kind of bike, from the expensive mountain bikes to the old large-tired kind or the sleeker small-tired type.

One big advantage to bike riding. If you have especially weak or hurting ankles, knees or hips, the bike is ready-made for you. The bike cuts to almost nothing the repetitive stress of your foot hitting the ground with each step. If you have lower back pain, again the bike may be your exercise tool of choice.

Now we come to the second advantage of biking. You can do it outside along residential streets or in parks or special bike paths. Or you can get the same result sitting in your living room watching TV or listening to a novel on tape on your stationary bike.

These are handy for several reasons: no traffic danger, no rain, snow or weather to worry about. Your air conditioner or heater keeps the temperature pleasant. You can catch up on your TV or taped novel at the same time you're exercising.

Cycling can do more than walking for some muscles. For example it builds up your thigh muscles. These help you stand and go up stairs and in lifting. Cycling also can strengthen the muscles around your knee joints. This can be a boon to those with knee pain.

Be sure to warm up gradually before serious bike work. This might be on your stationary by turning the resistance down to zero and just peddling away for five minutes with no strain. Outside, you might stay on flat surfaces for the first five minutes, not doing any hard riding.

Now the pains. If you hurt in your knees and lower back, take it easy on the bike inside or out. Outside, don't try to work up any hills and, inside, don't put on much resistance. Go the easy route for a week or two so your legs can built up strength to take on the new workload. Add tougher work as you get stronger. Listen to your body. It will tell you when you're ready to move on to the harder exercising.

SWIMMING & WATER EXERCISES

Exercising in water is a fairly new form of aerobic workout. The idea is to do simple body movements in shallow water—while the person is standing on the bottom of a pool and the water is at various levels from waist to shoulder height.

Exercising in water can be tough. Deeper water can mean the resistance to movement is as high as that with heavy free weights. Fibromyalgia patients must be cautious when doing water aerobics.

Talk with the instructor and learn what level of difficulty the routines are.

If they are minimal in resistance, they should work for you. Balance out your level of symptoms with the exercising need-ed and see if it fits. Working out in a heated pool gives several benefits besides the resistance factor. The warm water helps circulation and can give a high psychological boost as well. Exercises can also be done with flotation devices to aid the patient.

Swimming is said to be the most complete exercise that any one knows about. It works the most muscles in the body. It is low impact, the water holds up part of your weight, and a stroke such as the crawl or freestyle is the best for the quickest workout in a pool.

The one big drawback: you need a pool. Swimming in back yard pools is fine, but not the type of long distance workout you need. City pools, YMCAs, some hotel pools and motel pools are ideal for the long distance, lap after lap swimming.

Here, you should check out swimming with your doctor to be sure that it will not harm any of your FMS symptoms. If you get the green light, then pick your stroke, your difficulty level, and jump in. Or better, wade in and take it easy. Never swim when you are dizzy, feel ill or seem short of breath.

If you get tired, move at once to the side of the pool and get out or ask for help getting out. Drowning in three feet of water is not going to help your FMS.

BENEFITS OF WATER WORKOUTS

- Production of more serotonin and the growth hormone. These are big helps for most of the fibromyalgia problems.
- Improved lung capacity and strengthening of the heart muscles for better general health.
- Water support during exercises for those with some advanced fibromyalgia conditions.
- Water workouts promote better joint health partly because of the lack of stress compared to other exercises such as running and impact sports.
- A group exercise class in a pool is good for interaction with others. Can result in big social and emotional confidence.
- Stimulates the production of T-cells, which makes a stronger immune system, which helps the body fight off many FMS problems.
- Your movements in the water can help to cut down on stress and anxiety.
- Water workouts will bring more strength and flexibility for muscles and connective tissues in arms legs and shoulders. This is where many fibromyalgia problems

often develop.
• During the workouts, your muscles will be stimulated and then relax, which will help relieve their pain.

WEIGHT TRAINING

Now we come to a topic that is controversial for fibromyalgia patients. Here you definitely should talk to your doctor to see which types of weights and machines you can use safely. Depending on your particular FMS symptoms, you will have different routines than another fibromyalgia sufferer.

RESISTANCE BANDS

Your doctor will probably tell you that the best of all types of weight training are those done with a plastic band or tube. These are used extensively by physical therapists and often come in three strengths: yellow, red and green. The yellow is the weakest, and the green the strongest. Two brand names you might look for in a sports store are Thera-Band and Dynaband.

These plastic bands are used for direct pull, such as placing the ends of the band in your hand, forming a loop. Step on the loop's end and begin doing curl ups with your hand from waist to shoulder. To increase the resistance, wrap the band around your hand once. These can be tough workouts, yet do not threaten any damage to you that free weights can.

There are 50 different exercises you can do with an elastic band. It can be tied to a doorknob for straight pulls across your chest, behind your back and at your side. It can be used standing, sitting or lying down. There are manuals on the use of the stretch band, or a physical therapist can give you directions.

FREE WEIGHTS

If you have weights at home, or can borrow some, be sure to stick to the light side, five, ten or maybe fifteen pounds. Do your curl ups, over heads and side arm workouts, but be careful and get some professional help from a physical therapist to lay out a group of exercises you can do with your FMS limitations.

The same pattern follows on the use of machines in a gym or at home. Ask the attendants what you should be using and doing with your FMS. Explain the problem to them and see if they can help. If not, go to your physical therapist and if possible have that person tour the gym with you for his or her advice on which machines you can use safely.

As one last word, be careful with free weights and machines. It's very easy for the momentum of the weights to take you farther than you really wanted to go. The elastic band or tube is still the best exercise device in the strength field for you to use.

WHAT WEIGHT TRAINING WON'T DO

A lot of people, especially women, have a lot of wrong ideas about weight training, what it can and can't do. Here are some of the more prevalent old wives's tales about weight training and how wrong they are:

1. Working machines and lifting weights can spot reduce certain areas of your body like your hips or stomach. Not true. Exercise can help you reduce, but you reduce weight over your entire body, not one specific spot.
2. When you stop lifting weights, that muscle you generated will turn into fat. No way Jose. Any new muscle you have developed will only lose its size and tone, but if you're still eating as much as you did during training, those calories will turn into fat.
3. Weight lifting can pull muscles and break bones—it's dangerous. Nope. With good instruction and following the proper procedures and techniques, lifting is safe and can increase muscle mass and tone—and the work actually strengthens the bones to which those muscles are attached.
4. Weight lifting makes a woman bulky and inflexible. False. If you add a little muscle mass, you can then add in a stretching program as well to keep that new muscle flexible.
5. Women get huge muscles weight lifting and look more like men. Not unless they're trying to. Less testosterone

is produced by women than by men, so women build muscle much slower and smaller in size than a man would doing the same reps. Those huge men's muscles take years of hard work (four hours a day)—and in some cases dangerous steroids—to produce.

6. In strength training, much pain for any gain is the rule. Balderdash. Untrue. If your muscles are sore, you shouldn't be lifting. If your FMS has given you too many sore muscles, you probably should not lift at all. Consult with your doctor or your physical therapist.

7. Everyone starts with humongous heavy weights. Nuh-uh, lie, lie, lie. A beginner should start with a weight you can lift easily ten times (with the last two getting harder). For FMS patients this may be only one or two pounds. Others may start curl ups, say, with fifteen pounds. Depends on the individual. As you get stronger, over the months, you will want to go to gradually heavier weights.

CALORIE BURN-OFF

Yes, any kind of exercise is going to burn off some calories. For those of you interested in losing weight, here is a chart that shows in general terms just how much calorie burn you can expect from each kind of workout.

Exercise	Calorie burn in 15 minutes
Walking, 3 mph	65
Walking, 4 mph	100
Walking up stairs	150
Walking up hills	125
Aerobic Dancing	100
Bicycling, 6 mph	70
Bicycling, 10 mph	105
Stationary Bike, moderate	70
Running, 12 min/mile	143
Running, 8 min/mile	215
Running, 6 min/mile	260
Nordic Track Machine	150

Swimming, crawl stroke	145
Stair Climber machine	155
Treadmill, moderate speed	120

CHAPTER 8

STRETCHING

Y ou see runners do it before a race. You see ballet dancers do it before a show. You see football and baseball players do it before every game. It's called stretching and in effect it helps the body get ready for the exercising that is to come.

Stretching is not warming up. Many experts say you should warm up before you stretch. This might include a brief walk, some side straddle hops or body twists and another walk. When you feel warmed up, then is the time to do some serious stretching.

For people with FMS, stretching is a vital part of any type of exercise program. No matter what you do for your exercise workout, do a warm-up and stretching first.

Many people with fibromyalgia sit around all day, don't get up and move or be active. The pain is less that way. The only problem is the pain is never going to lessen by sitting around.

Lack of motion, let alone exercise, lets the muscles and ligaments lose their flexibility, tone and strength. There goes the old ball game.

Flexibility for most FMS patients tends to be impaired in the lower back and neck, shoulders, hips and thighs.

Stretching usually works best if done after your aerobic workout. It's a good way to cool down. Stretching is most effective if you do it every day. If you exercise six days a week, be sure to do your stretching cool down every day.

Here are some other stretching tips:

STRETCH EVERY DAY. Don't stretch before your exercise or use it as a warm-up. Your warm-up can be a short walk, or some easy calisthenics like arm swings, neck and trunk rotation. Most anything like this to get your blood pumping faster than normal.

DO YOUR STRETCHING SLOWLY. Don't bounce or press too hard. A slow, easy stretch should be felt, but not to the point of pain. Pain means you may have pulled the muscle instead of just stretching it. When a muscle is stretched slowly and evenly, there should be no pain and no contraction of the muscle. Hold a gentle stretch for five or six seconds. If you've done it right the muscle will relax a little and you can stretch it a little more. Hold this one for ten seconds, then release it gently and return to the original position.

CONCENTRATE ON THE MUSCLE YOU'RE STRETCHING. Don't think about the rent coming due, or the kids or the state of your marriage. Work on the muscle now; do the rest later.

START YOUR RELAXATION PROGRAM WITH THE EASIEST OF THE STRETCHING ROUTINES. Some samples come later.

Progress and results of your stretching will come slowly. Don't overdo it and don't give up. Keep at it and you'll find that it pays off. No, you won't be able to do the splits and a ballet jump, but the stretching should help your pain level reduce. Try to do these stretches on a thick carpet or exercise pad.

SPECIAL STRETCHES FOR FMS PATIENTS

Yes, we're here to the nitty-gritty. These stretching procedures are especially designed to help those with fibromyalgia. We stretch the muscles that hurt the most: that includes those in the neck, upper back, shoulders, arms, lower back, hips and the hamstrings in back of the thighs. Utilize these stretches:

1. FOR YOUR LOWER BACK AND HIPS:

Lie on your back with your arms extended level with your

shoulders. Lift your left leg as high as you can, vertical if possible, and then turn your body and bring down your left foot and put it on your right hand. If it won't go all the way, bring your hand up to meet the foot.

Now, stretch your foot toward your hand for five seconds, relax for a few seconds and then stretch your foot downward again. You should get a little farther this time. Repeat three times. Then return the leg to the floor and do the same stretch with the right foot to the left hand. Do three times.

2. FOR YOUR LOWER BACK AND BUTTOCKS:

Lie on your back on the floor keeping your hands beside your body, legs out straight and feet together. Bring both knees toward your chest slowly. This will stretch your lower back and buttocks. Hold for ten seconds and return to starting position. Repeat the stretch four times.

3. FOR YOUR SHOULDERS, UPPER BACK MUSCLES AND THE TRUNK ROTATORS:

Sit on the floor and cross your legs, pulling your feet as close to your buttocks as possible. Now twist to the right with your trunk and both arms. Go as far as you can, then grab the left arm with your right hand and pull it even farther to the right. This will stretch your upper arm, back and shoulder. Hold this for ten seconds, then release gently and return facing front. Repeat this stretch three times to the right, then do it three times to the left.

4. FOR YOUR LOWER BACK MUSCLES, HIP FLEXORS AND HAMSTRINGS:

Lie on your back with your legs fully extended and feet together, your hands by your sides. Pull up your right knee to your chest, and keep the other leg extended. Put both hands under the right knee and pull the leg toward your chest for a gentle stretch. Hold the position for ten seconds and return leg to the floor. Do this three times, then repeat with the other leg.

5. FOR YOUR HAMSTRINGS, LOWER BACK AND BUTTOCKS:

While sitting on the floor with your legs straight in front of you, extend your arms forward and reach toward your toes as far as you can without pain. This will put a gentle stretch on your hamstrings, your lower back and your buttocks. When you have reached as far as possible in a gentle move, hold it for ten seconds. After ten seconds return to the position you started. Do this four or five times, trying to stretch a little farther each time. Don't over do it, and don't lunge or bounce.

6. FOR YOUR NECK, YOUR UPPER BACK AND YOUR CHEST:

For this one, stand behind a kitchen type chair. Place both your hands on the back of the chair. Now move back until your hands are still on the chair and your upper torso is parallel with the floor. Now bend your torso lower toward the floor letting your head come between your arms. After ten seconds in this position, lower your head even more so you can look back at your legs. This will give a gentle stretch to your neck muscles. After ten seconds here, move easily back to the starting position. Work this stretch five times.

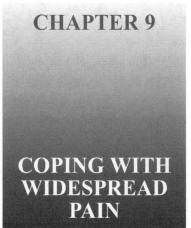

CHAPTER 9

COPING WITH WIDESPREAD PAIN

It's a fact: coping with widespread pain is the toughest part of having fibromyalgia. It's a challenge for many with it just to get out of bed in the morning. They know that there is going to be another day of pain, deep seated, perhaps in several parts of their body, chronic and at the same time unpredictable. It's enough to get even the strongest willed person down in the dumper. That can lead to depression—and then the FMS patient has a whole new set of problems.

So how do you cope with the pain?

As you know, there is no known cure for fibromyalgia. There is no immediate hope in that direction. That means each person has to develop a strategy, a system, a plan for coping with his or her individual set of FMS pains.

Some people say that to feel secure they don't have to be in control of everything, but they do want to feel that their lives are at least organized. For the FMS patient that can be important too—and it comes down to a plan to fight your pain. Some medical folks call it pain management. The idea is to set up a battlefield plan and work your plan and win at least some of the time. Here are some of the strategies that your army can try that work for many people.

FOOL YOUR BRAIN

Your brain gets all kinds of stimuli all day, every waking second through your five senses. One that it gets from FMS patients is that of pain. A method that you can use to confuse your nerve signals is to send other signals to the brain with the idea of excluding or dampening the severity of the pain signal.

Are you with me? This can be done by thinking about the most pleasant time you ever had. That might be when you first fell in love, or when you were proposed to. Maybe your honeymoon or the first time you received a really good promotion at work. You're tricking your brain by sending it all sorts of pleasant memory signals, and that nasty old pain signal gets lost in the bunch and never gets through with its full power.

Psychologically this is sound, and can be used for many things besides pain. It works well for any kind of bad news/bad situation. Give it a try on your FMS pains. Happy thoughts.

The same idea works by doing other pleasurable things, like talking with your best friend about happy things, taking a hot bath, watching a funny movie. Remember that laughing is also good for your FMS. Do something pleasurable that you thoroughly enjoy—maybe a hobby, or gardening, or writing a happy, up-beat letter to a friend.

USE YOUR IMAGINATION

Technically this is called guided imagery and there are commercial books and tapes how to do it. Briefly, most of them use a pleasant voice and soft music to help you imagine a gentle, soft place where you can feel at peace. If you can get caught up in this fairyland place, it can lull you into relaxation that will, for a few hours, wipe out how you feel your pain. It will still be there, but you simply won't be aware of it. This type of total relaxation should also help reduce the muscle tightness in your neck and shoulders, and promote overall body muscle relaxation. This method of fighting pain may last for only two or three hours. The more you utilize this guided imagery the longer the effects will last.

PSYCH YOURSELF DOWN AND RELAX

The word relaxation has been used several times so far. This is one of the keys in fighting your pain. The more relaxed you are, the better you can cope with the pain. When you get stressed and uptight you're lighting a fire under your pain and zooming it right over the moon.

Have you heard of relaxation exercises? Look in bookstores or maybe a large music store for products that promote relaxation exercises. If you can put yourself into a state of deep relaxation with these aids, that will help your muscles loosen up—and that means they will be less painful.

What will those relaxation exercise books tell you to do? Here is a sample from one of them. Take a look. Give it a try:

WARMING YOURSELF

You'll need a comfortable chair in a spot where no one will bother you for at least ten minutes. Go through the exercise trying as hard as you can to follow the instructions and the words.

First, close both eyes and think about your left arm. Now open your eyes and read these words slowly, with emphasis.

...I need to relax all of the muscles in my left arm.
...Relax them, now.
Pause for ten seconds, relaxing your arm.
...I am now letting all of those arm muscles relax.
...Relax them, let them go limp and restful.
Pause for ten seconds, still relaxing your left arm.
...Now I have control of my left arm and I will push all of the tension and tightness out of my arm.
...Push it out, push it out now.
Pause for ten seconds, still pushing out the tensions.
...My left arm feels heavy; it is heavy and warm.
Pause for ten seconds.
...My left arm is much heavier now, much heavier.
Pause for five seconds.
...Now my left arm feels much warmer and much heavier.
Pause for five seconds.

...Each time I breathe, my arm feels warmer, heavier, and like it is so relaxed that it will never hurt again.

Now, go through the same procedure for your right arm, then for both of your legs—one at a time.

That's the pattern. Go over it until you can recite it from memory, and then keep your eyes closed during the whole exercise on all four areas. Did it work? Do your limbs feel looser, less tense? It may take two or three sessions to get this to work. Try the other relaxation exercises in the book.

Cold Can Help

Some people—both FMS patients and others—say that they can find help for painful areas by using cold instead of the usual heat.

The idea is that cold slows everything down, from electricity in your battery, to sound traveling through cold air, to nerve impulses going from painful muscles to the old brain.

By using cold packs, cold cloths, ice packs, or even a plastic bag of frozen peas from your freezer, you might be able to cut into that pain and slow it down a little. Frozen peas? Right, they are small and the bag is pliable and can be used to bend around a joint or flow over a larger area. When they unfreeze, toss them back in and freeze them again. Oh, you probably shouldn't plan on eating these often-refrozen peas. Put a big X on the package. Be careful with cold. You can get a burn from ice going directly on the bare skin for too long. It looks like frostbite and is serious.

Heat? Yes, it works

As we have said in other chapters, heat can be used to help reduce pain in muscles and around joints, and to simply make your whole body feel better. Nothing like a hot shower. We know that heat on the body increases the blood flow through the surface areas, and that pumps it around faster through the whole body. Here you can use a little psychology on yourself. As that heat is going into your body, tell yourself that each moment it is relaxing your muscles more and more and they hurt less and less.

How do you get this heat? Several ways. Pick out your favorite or try them all:

Hot tub or shower tops the list. Then come moist heating pads, whirlpool hot tubs, warm swimming pools, hot towels, moist hot hydro packs, heated mattress pads and blankets, electric heating pads, infrared heating lamps, microwave gel packs.

SELF-HYPNOSIS

Hypnosis is a rather controversial method for putting a person into a deep relaxing sleep. It is best used by a qualified—and in some states a registered and licensed—hypnotherapist. Some say it's dangerous to put a patient in the hands of another person where post-hypnotic suggestions can trigger actions in the person well after the session is over. Proponents say that no one will do anything in response to a post-hypnotic suggestion that they wouldn't do while awake and normal.

Self-hypnosis can be learned by most people from a qualified hypnotist. It is a way to go into a totally relaxed state where no pain will bother you. You can also learn to give yourself post-hypnotic suggestions that can help alter your behavior in regards to your constant pain. If you're interested, ask your doctor to suggest a qualified hypnotherapist.

BIOFEEDBACK

We talked about this before. It can help manage your intense pain. It works on the pain management centers to produce deep muscle relaxation and give you relief. Here you will need direction, and treatment and instruction. But then you will be able to utilize the principles of biofeedback you have learned to help you to cope with your pain.

EXERCISE

This was covered extensively in a previous chapter. Just remember that it's one of the best ways to help reduce pain and to get yourself back into the flow of life. Aerobic exercises, especially, are good. They release endorphins, the body's natural pain relievers.

Bike riding, walking, swimming, roller blading, all help get more oxygen to your muscles. You should continue less strenuous exercises even during painful periods. You'll want to reduce the time and difficulty of the workout. Stretching, again limited, is still good to do during pain flare-ups.

MEDICATIONS

Many kinds of medications are used by most FMS patients to manage pain. Be sure that you have gone over all of your daily medications with your doctor. Also ask what ones you need to increase when you have a serious pain flare-up.

CHANGING SLEEP PATTERNS

Many times when there is increased pain it is the result of a change in your sleep pattern. Maybe you are sleeping less, your deep sleep is not deep enough, or you simply are not getting the required right kind of sleep to help your body function correctly.

The reduced sleep can cut down the amount of serotonin in your body, and that alone can cause more pain.

The answer may be a simple adjustment of the dosage of some of your medications. It could be your mate is snoring. This is an easy one: use earplugs or move to another room. Sometimes back pain will cut down your restful sleep. One way to combat this is to have an adjustable bed. Move it so your body is in the best position to relieve your back pain. You might try to sleep on a reclining chair. If your own snoring is keeping you awake, the earplugs are great. They cut out 35% of exterior noise and should let you slumber away the night.

Managing your pain and the flare-ups is a highly personal job. Try different things and find out what works best for you. Then have those items handy so you can use them when the time comes. Have gel packs for heat and cold, frozen peas, a supply of earplugs. You may find that a non-caffeine soft drink helps or warm milk before bedtime. Use your best exercise method or the hot shower or swimming and walking. Know what will work for you under different situations. Have your ammunition ready for a flare-up attack at any time and then counter-attack with a vengeance.

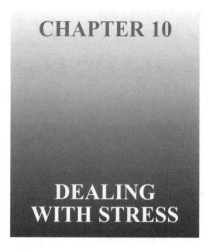

CHAPTER 10

DEALING WITH STRESS

I t is entirely normal to be stressed when pain forces you to give up many of your activities, makes your everyday household routines nearly impossible and the pain constantly touches you all day whether you're working, sitting, standing or trying to get to sleep. Stress is murder.

WHAT IS STRESS?

Stress has been described as the response of your mind, emotions and your body to the work-a-day world and all the pressures of modern life. Actual events are not stress. It is our reactions and our emotional response to those events that brings us stress.

Doctors see stress or the lack of it every day. One patient may become highly stressed and even depressed when she breaks a leg and must give up tennis for six weeks. Another woman who also plays tennis takes a broken leg in stride, and spends the time studying films of great tennis players, talking with her coach how to improve her own game, and doing referee work on the high chair during club matches.

Fibromyalgia patients fall into the same general pattern. About a third of FMS patients are highly stressed by the symptoms of this syndrome. Another third are normally stressed by the problems. Then there is a third who are less stressed than normal by FMS.

YOUR OWN STRESS GAUGE

No matter how well you can handle your FMS symptoms, sooner or later they will get to you. Here are some of the sign-posts of being over-stressed:

1. Nausea
2. Anxiety
3. Irritability
4. Loss of appetite
5. Painful muscle tension
6. Excess nervousness
7. Fatigue
8. Sweaty hands

When stress strikes, it becomes a part of a dangerous cycle.

Stress in the extreme can lead to a shock of the body and a weaker immune system. This can make your FMS symptoms worse: more pain, less sleep, more agitation. This will result in more stress, and that leads to a weaker immune system…the cycle goes on and on.

Do you see where this is going? The mind must work with the body to produce stress. The experts tell us that stress affects the body's immune system, the autonomic nervous system and the endocrine system. Some big words but they are all true. It's the mind and body working together—in this case to hurt the body.

When we look at fibromyalgia, many say that stress happens not from huge problems and tragedies. Rather it comes as a result of those frustrating and annoying little daily situations and hassles that we all have. These myriad causes of stress are magnified when there is little support of family, co-workers, friends, and sometimes even a physician who doesn't understand what FMS is all about.

TAKE A SURVEY OF YOUR STRESS LEVEL

Stress is much more a problem and much more serious than most people and physicians will admit. Stress is all around us every day. In this modern world we have hundreds of things to worry about that our farmer ancestors on the plains of Nebraska never even knew about.

The Industrial Revolution saw to that. The modern day electronic revolution has super-psyched us up into multi billion bytes of problems and concerns and worries that many of us are simply not quite ready to understand, let alone accept.

A survey recently told us that nearly a hundred million Americans have at least one stress-caused problem and take medication for it. Some doctors say that as much as 80 percent of all illness that physicians see every day is stress-induced. That is quite an indictment of our society. This is to let you know that you are not alone in this stressful situation while evaluating your own stress profile.

One good thing about this little personal mini-survey you're going to do. It might help you pinpoint certain activities, acquaintances, or even friends who turn up your stress quotient into the billion mega watt level. So, dump a friend? Quit the bowling league where the best bowler on the team gives you hives every Tuesday night when he criticizes your bowling form? Who knows? Take a look at the survey below and have some answers for yourself. Do any of these situations give you trouble?

- hostility
- too much sleep
- too little sleep
- caregiving to a dependent person
- repressed feelings
- negative attitude
- loneliness
- job problems
- depression
- problems communicating
- bad diet
- feeling of worthlessness
- no real exercise
- no job, few prospects

- death of a loved one
- divorce
- separation
- can't quit smoking
- addiction to medications
- alcoholic
- use of illegal drugs
- over-involved in environmental issues

Did some of those areas of activity hit home? You may want to take another long look at that list. Is there some problem or situation there that you could phase out of your every day life to help make it less stressful? Hey, nobody said this would be easy. Maybe you should go back with a different colored pen and mark areas of concern on the list you need to consider again.

How Can You Tell if You're Over-stressed?

Fibromyalgia is sneaky. You don't need to be told that. So is stress. It can crop up from two dozen different reasons. The big problem is that it can be hit-or-miss, and can affect one person seriously and leave the next one pink cheeked and laughing. Which of these stress symptoms crank up your stress thermometer?

- feelings of doom
- headaches
- anger
- dry mouth
- back pain
- unhappiness
- racing heart
- boredom
- anxiety
- dizziness
- sweating palms
- bossiness
- ears ringing
- grinding teeth

- lots of body aches, pains
- problems sleeping
- worrying constantly
- forgetfulness
- bowel or bladder changes
- restlessness
- cry easily
- memory loss
- no sense of humor
- loneliness
- not the usual creativity
- dizziness
- compulsive eating
- can't make decisions
- indigestion
- light-headedness
- use more drugs, alcohol, cigarettes.

Now with your check on certain items above, you can start to manage your stress level. Hey, are you too bossy around others? Think about it. If it's true, you can make a conscious decision not to be so bossy. You can ease back in a situation, let someone else take the lead, let them be bossy, and watch your stress level ease off.

Pick out half-a-dozen of the above stress points that you can work on. It won't come all in a day, but the more of them you can counter, and subjugate or eliminate, the easier your life will be and the lower your stress—which should also mean a lowering of your symptoms of FMS.

No-Control Stress

Yes, there are a lot of events in your life you have little or no control over. These also are the ones that can zoom your stress level right off the charts. Here are the ten happenings in a person's life that create the greatest impact on the stress level. These are listed in order of intensity of impact on most people:

Death of a spouse. Divorce. Marriage. Marital separation. A jail term. Death of a close family member other than spouse.

Severe personal injury or illness. Fired from your job. Retirement. Pregnancy. Difficulties in sexual performance.

If one of these high-stress events happens to you, be sure to get some help, look at the situation and see how you can reduce the stress it brings. Knowing how tough it is going to be will be a big help. This goes for any of the forty or fifty high stress events in your life. Be ready. Know how to meet them. Plan ahead.

CAN STRESS EVER BE POSITIVE?

Absolutely it can. Say you get a big bonus at work—a raise and a corner office. You call your wife or husband with the news and almost fly home. Your energy level is bumping the ceiling. You feel great. Your body has just supplied you with enough adrenaline to keep you going for a week. Besides just feeling good, this type of positive stress can help you down the road, make you like your job better, get along with others, and help you for months.

Yet, there is always a way to turn a positive stress like this into a negative. Say a grandmother has just received the good news: 7 pounds 8 ounces and 21 inches long, a new baby boy. The grandmother is thrilled but gets into a dither worrying about how she's going to be able to make the travel connections. She gets so upset and sick that she decides not to make the trip.

WHAT MAKES YOUR STRESS WORSE?

Almost anything you don't like doing, don't want to do, are afraid to do or just hate to do will accentuate your stress quotient.

Like what? Like asking your boss for a raise. Like misplacing or losing things. Like going into a room to do something and forgetting why you went.

It might be as simple as waiting in traffic for a light to change. Being caught in a traffic jam on the freeway. Going out to dinner with friends. Entertaining friends at home. Getting ready for a holiday. Having to make choices. Fear of rejection by family or fellow workers.

It could also be: Coping with everyday family situations at home. Working with people who annoy you. Painting a room. Worrying about your fibromyalgia. Being short on money to pay bills. A problem with your spouse. Slowing of your sexual powers. Waiting in line at a bank or grocery store.

Some people—even with fibromyalgia—can do many of the above things and not have them produce stress. Others might turn and run from each one of them, and in the very act make their symptoms of FMS worse.

Even if some of these have bugged you in the past, now is the time to turn it around. How? Say you're waiting in line at the post office. Instead of drumming your fingers on the counter, take along a good mystery to read as you wait. No stress, no worry about the passing time, and you'll get into the mystery. Try a similar change of emphasis this way on other stress situations.

First you have to recognize those activities that drive you up the wall. Sit down, right now, and make a list of them. How many? Fifteen, twenty, four? Get them all down and look at them. How can you detour around these problems or figure out ways to reduce their impact on your life? The traffic waits? Hey, see if you can go to work an hour earlier. That might get you out of the worst of the traffic jams mornings, and go home an hour earlier at night. Figure a counter-punch for each of your high stress terror points.

Yes, it will take some time, some thought. But if you can work it out for even half of them, you'll cut down on your stress, and that should slow down some of the fibromyalgia problems. At least those troubles won't get worse because of your stress.

SOME GENERAL GUIDELINES FOR STRESS REDUCTION

Have you seen a sheet of paper that has a form for the week and lines to list all of your commitments for that coming week? This is a great idea. If you don't have the form, make a list for each day of the coming week. Put down everything you are scheduled to do.

Church choir on Thursday night. Take kids to Little League on Tuesday and Friday at 3:30. Bowling on Tuesday at noon. Doctor's appointment on Friday at 9 a.m. Laundry on Monday. Clean house on Saturday. Ballet classes Monday and Wednesday. List all you have set to do that week, for both day and night, work and play, in and out of the house.

Now, look it over. Any conflicts? Have you allowed enough time to get each job done before the next one is due? You might want to kick in another fifteen minutes for each project so you don't get a speeding ticket making your next meeting.

Now, look at your "calendar" in general. Are you simply trying to do too much? Have you over-committed? Do you have to do the program once every month for your women's meeting? Is it time for you to evaluate your schedule and see where you can cut back? This might be mandatory if the pain and fatigue from your FMS flares up and knocks you down for a day or a week. Always have a fire escape in case you need to have someone else take your place or do the work you thought you had to. Here is where friends are a prime factor. They will help. Ask them.

You have to learn just how much you can do in your current FMS situation. This will increase and decrease with your pain and fatigue and sleep problems. By monitoring yourself, and evaluating your activities, you should be able to bring down your stress level and that in turn we hope will lessen the severity of your FMS pains.

Yes, when you set down your schedule, you may find that there are some of your activities that aren't all that important to you or your family. You may want to take a critical look at these and perhaps slim down your workload, by bowing out of some groups or organizations that don't mean that much to you. That will help leave more time for the important things like quality family time.

A Day Person or a Night Person?

The secret here is not to be a twelve-hours-a-day worker. Don't work all day and then keep working to midnight every day. Don't work seven days a week for months on end. This will quickly zoom your stress right over the moon.

If you have too much work to get done at the office, have a talk with your boss. Explain your FMS and its limitations. Explain that if you keep on your overworked schedule you might be down and out for a month or two. Show him or her that an 8 hour day will be best for both of you.

If you work for yourself, especially at home as more and more people are these days, be stern with yourself. Don't work too long. Take time off for family, for fun, and for the future.

Say your pain is better in the afternoons than the mornings. At your job, schedule your meetings and conferences in the afternoons when you will be at your best. It helps.

Do What You Can Do

A young man was a promising marathon runner. Then he was in a car wreck that paralyzed both his legs. He was devastated. He knew he could never run another marathon. Then he remembered seeing people in wheelchairs doing marathons. He could do that. He did. Became a local celebrity and talked to wheelchair-bound kids and older people, encouraging them to do all they could do.

The same thing holds for FMS patients. You have to do all you can do. You might never run a marathon, but you can get off your bottom and get back to walking around the block every day. There are lots of things you can do. What about reading to kids at your local school? Helping slow readers to learn to read better? Getting up and around and figuring out just what you can do around the house and what you can't do—for right now?

Trying to be perfect can stress out anyone. For an FMS patient just trying to do everything to perfection will shoot your stress level up a dozen notches. You don't have to serve excellent meals every time. You don't have to keep your house spotless, the laundry done every day on time, or be the best clerk or secretary or manager on your job. Do the best you can and be happy with that. There will be days when your pains and your fatigue drag you down. Work though it as best you can and hope for a better, calmer, tomorrow.

STRESS ELIMINATION

Something was said earlier about naming your stress factors and trying to eliminate them. Now we do it in earnest. Make out a list of the people, things, actions and events that really get your dander up. This list might also include work and relatives.

Now you have a list of stress factors. Are there any that you can simply eliminate? How about that Thursday night pinochle game? It used to be fun. You knew everyone well, friends of long standing. Then it changed. New people came in, others dropped out. Now there are two women in the group who simply drive you over the mountain. Drop out. Give it up. Reduce one level of stress.

Think of any parts of your life that you can change with little loss, and eliminate a stress point. You may have to learn to say no. You can't be the PTA chairman this year. No, you can't possibly run the concession stand at two little league baseball games a week.

Tip: When you say no, always have the name of another person to suggest who might do it.

Are there any of your stresses that you can downplay and learn to manage? This might be a person who really riles you at work. Can you shift your job a little or work with another person of the same level to get the work done? Try to avoid contact with that person and thereby cut out a stress problem.

Go back over your list. Are there any more points you need to add that increase your stress quotient? If so put them down. You can't do everything at once. Pick out one or two of them that you've known you should straighten out for some time, and get those done. Then move on to the other ones.

You're going to be glad you did. Your stress level should come down and that should let you get more and better sleep and that should help with lowering, rather than increasing your FMS symptoms.

STRESS ON THE JOB

By its very nature, fibromyalgia creates a lot of problems when you work outside the house. With your fatigue and pain alone, there are more than enough big problems that can cause all sorts of added stress on the job. Because this is such a big topic, we're going to devote a whole chapter to it later.

EVER KEPT A DAILY JOURNAL?

More and more people these days are keeping daily journals—notes and thoughts and ideas and a record of what happened that day. This is a good discipline for anyone, and it can be especially beneficial for fibromyalgia patients.

Too often we keep our hopes and fears bottled up inside somewhere so no one can find out about them. FMS patients tend to do this more than others. So the daily journal is one place you can be completely honest. Tell your journal exactly how you feel. It hurts, damnit, and you hate it. It hurts and you're tired all the time and you can't sleep and you don't know what you're going to do.

Once it's down on paper for the first time, or the tenth time, you can be more aware of it, and start to figure out just how you can get along with your problems, and at the same time learn how to try to lessen them.

One of the benefits of a journal is simple record keeping. You can plot out the cycles of your pain and fatigue. Is there a pattern? Is there any reason that such a pattern should exist? Say you're having trouble sleeping. You keep mentioning it in your journal. When you check back a few weeks later, and see the pattern of your sleep problems, you may be able to tie that in with some emotional situation at the time, or some other trigger that set off your sleeplessness. It gives you a handle on how you might be able to prevent such a sleep situation in the future. Avoid the trigger that caused the flare-up.

A daily journal is also a wonderful way to develop your writing ability. Say you do your stint every day on the computer. You do a single spaced page. That's quite a bit of writing. And it will nudge you into thinking more and more about your previous day, and what you did, what you didn't get done, what you dream of doing and what you want to do today. You might even include a MUST DO list for that day or the next one. Think about it. A daily journal is great to look back on after six months. An easy way is to print them out on your computer, three hole punch them and put them in a three ring binder.

CAN YOU TALK TO PEOPLE?

Being able to communicate with family and friends and co-workers is one of the basics of human conduct. Too often a chronic disease like fibromyalgia dampens down that skill as you wrestle with your constant pain, frustration, fatigue, lack of sleep and general damnit-to-hell feeling.

When you should be talking out some small problem with your kids, you are in the middle of a flare-up of pain and hassling with the kids is the last thing you can do. Sometimes a put-off gets to be a forgotten item. Try to work through the basic and necessary communications you need to do with family, friends and workers. This will take a lot of concentration on your part, a "playing with pain" syndrome that pro athletes get used to. You'll have to get used to doing it too.

As a last resort, you may want to ask for some psychological counseling to learn new ways to communicate through your pain. True, it won't be easy, and it won't come quickly, but it will be worth it.

BE COOL

This is a slang phrase that has been in the language for fifty years. It just won't go away. It's also a great phrase to use in the way you look at the problems that rear up constantly, and with your pain and frustration. Hey, be cool. If the problem looks like it is earth shattering, ease off, think about it, don't do a sudden knee-jerk reaction. Hey, be cool.

Try to think through some problem or frustration and put it in the right perspective. It just isn't as bad as it looked. This, too, will pass. Be cool. Hey, you can handle this. Yeah, you can take this in stride and come out a winner. Don't balloon those little ones into big ones that will magnify your stress and hurt you even more. Okay, so let's just be cool.

STIMULANTS YOU DON'T NEED

NICOTINE: A drug, a stimulant to the central nervous system that can give you a boost, and at the same time can surge your stress quotient right out the window. You don't need that. Non-smokers have fewer bouts with stress than those who smoke a pack a day. You don't need it.

HARD DRUGS: Dozens of different kinds that do various bad things to your body. You don't need the drug problem to add to your FMS symptoms, and in the long run they will make all of your hurts that much more hurtful. One problem at a time is best.

CAFFEINE: You bet, another drug you don't need. True, it can perk you up for a time, but it then will let you down with a whump, and you'll be feeling more pain than you did before. One of the big problems with caffeine is that it increases the blood pressure and heart rate, and worst of all it can make you as nervous as a long tailed cat in a room filled with people moving back and forth in their rocking chairs. What has caffeine? You know: coffee, cola products, tea and even a chocolate bar. A good cup of coffee will run you 125 mg of caffeine. Tea up to 100 mg, a Coke or Pepsi is 45 mg and that chocolate bar is only 2 mg. Have a chocolate instead of that coffee.

STRESS AND YOU

Yes, you're right. We've given you a lot to think about and a lot to do in this chapter on stress. That's because it's one of the basic factors you can use to actively fight your FMS. Reducing your stress is going to make a big difference in your every day life. We hope you can simplify it, cut down on extraneous activities, concentrate on what you feel you must do, and then have time left over to work on new ways to reduce your stress and your pain. Get at it.

CHAPTER 11

BATTLING YOUR FATIGUE

Fatigue on a daily and continuing basis is one of the worst aspects of fibromyalgia. Everyone has it. Everyone tries to fight against it. Few succeed. It's frustrating, debilitating. But it is one aspect of FMS that you can actively do something about.

You know the drill. Your day may start out as not the best. You know that you have a limited amount of energy. And you know you have to be selective how you use it. Here are some ways to help you ration out your reserves to get the most out of them and out of your day.

MAKE A LIST

Put down in a list what you need to do today. Don't worry about the rest of the week or the month. Concentrate on today.

Is this the usual list of things you regularly do? If so, are there any items that you can cancel or postpone or move around to another day?

Are there too many activities on your list? Can you simply cut down on your overall activities? If you have kids, there are a lot of trips and meetings and practices that must be done. Maybe you can start a car pool with a neighbor to get your kids to the games. Then you drive every other game.

Can you group your errands? Cut down on trips?

Now with your reduced list, reschedule your items so you do the toughest things during your high energy level time. Answer mail, pay bills, etc. at your lower energy times.

CUT IT OUT

You made your list and it's still too long. Even after you selected three things to say no to. Cut out some things you could do routinely in the past. This is now. Accept your limitations. Now concentrate on cutting down on your workload. Buy clothes you don't have to iron. Grocery shop once every two weeks and plan ahead and buy ahead. Eliminate every energy draining activity that you do not have to do. Every little bit helps.

YOUR OWN TOP TEN LIST

Back to that list you made of activities, meetings, etc. Take another look at the skinned down group. Now your job is to make out your top ten list. Rank these activities in order of importance to you. Give them numbers from one to ten or how many you have on the list.

With this weighted group in hand you can decide which items have the most importance and benefit. Be sure you get those done first, maybe some of the others can wait until tomorrow or until you are feeling stronger.

You might want to write that list on a 3 x 5 card and put it in your pocket—and keep it with you. If your memory sags to peanuts in the afternoon, a look at your priority card will help keep you on track. It might even include a short nap—add one on if you need it.

THE GARAGE SALE MOVE

Just moving around a big chair that you really don't need can turn into an energy-draining chore when your fatigue kicks in. Take a look at your place. How much "stuff" do you have lying around there that gets in the way and you really don't need?

Most of us hang onto things we've long since grown away from or out of. It might be furniture, clothing, tools, kitchen appliances and even pots and pans. Ever think of having a yard sale? Get together everything you don't want and don't need and put an ad in the newspaper.

To do this best, make an insurance inventory of everything in your house. Bet you haven't done that. Do this on a day you have lots of energy. It's a task. Now look over the inventory list and start whacking out things you should put out for the yard/garage sale.

You'll be surprised. You'll find things you didn't even know you still had.

Look at the inventory again. Could things in your house be better grouped or organized? All bedding in one place, all clothes in another, picture albums and old letters in a box plainly labeled. Try to organize things so you can find what you want when you need it. This will cut down a batch of work and make it easier to cope on one of those high fatigue days.

Take a look at your closets. Now there can be a gold mine of unwanted items. Most closets could be better set up and organized as well. In the end it will mean less work for you in your day-by-day living with your FMS pain and fatigue.

DELEGATION OF WORK

Remember when you used to have the kids help out? You delegated certain chores to them: dishes, setting the table, moving the lawn, cleaning their rooms. Good times.

The idea of delegating duties still holds no matter how old or young you are. If you don't have to do a job, think how much energy you are saving.

Back to your list of activities. Pick out one or two items that you might be able to delegate, then work on it. Do you have a friend who could go to the grocery store for you to do your shopping? Give her a list and some cash and she's off.

Maybe you have some mail to send but can't get up energy to go to the branch post office just three blocks away. A neighbor might be going that way. Call him and ask. Chances are he will be glad to run your package to the mailbox even if he was not headed that way.

If you are hurting so much that you simply can't get all of your housework done, it's probably time to call in a hired hand to help. The wash, the cleaning, vacuuming and scrubbing the kitchen floor can be done by a helper once a week and keep your place spic and span. The cost isn't that great. The dividends are tremendous.

When you're having a bad day or a bad week, don't get down on yourself because you can't do everything that you used to do. This bad time will pass and it will get better. Work toward reducing your stress and conserving your energy during high fatigue periods.

MAKE PEAK ENERGY TIMES COUNT

Let's say you are having a hard time sleeping, with the result that you run out of gas by two o'clock every afternoon. That means that you need to shift your important work and activity time to the morning when your energy level is higher.

Set up morning meetings instead of afternoon ones. Have a power breakfast instead of dinner with a client or co-worker. Set up your exercise time for morning, maybe do the shopping then if you're at home, and get the household things done that must be done before the blahs set in.

If your spouse is available, morning sex will be much better than a try late at night when you are too exhausted to participate.

There is a meeting or a party that you don't want to miss. How do you handle this? If you have the time and place, set up an hour-long nap before the event. Psychologists say we often are the sharpest just after we have had a brain time-out like a nap.

Now, even though you are having a low energy period, try your best not to let that control your life. Fight back by smiling more, telling good jokes, and trying your best to enjoy life. For balance, you might want to think of a friend who is confined to a wheelchair or a hospital bed. Think how many good things you really have.

Set Up a Schedule

Okay, that list again. You know what you have to do today. The most important are named first, and you're working down the priorities. Now, what you need to do is to schedule yourself so you have some time between those jobs to relax a moment and catch your breath. Pace yourself like an athlete.

If halfway through the afternoon you really bomb out and can't get out of your chair, you're still ahead. You finished your most important things already—the rest can wait until tomorrow.

If you set up a schedule like this for every day, you'll find that you will get more done, and still have time to play and be with your family and enjoy life. By pacing yourself for all week, you'll see that you don't wipe out on Wednesday and waste the week trying to recuperate. Give it a try. Schedule, pace, rest.

Sleep

The greatest fatigue fighter every FMS patient has is sleep. The more restful, deep sleep you can get, the better you will feel and the less severe all of your symptoms will be. Sleep is the key, and we have devoted a full chapter to it later on. For better sleep, you may need to take a look at your medications and talk it over with your doctor. Some adjustments and changes in meds may be needed.

Take a good long look at the chapter on sleep.

CHAPTER 12

DEPRESSION AND YOU

Depression is another problem for many of you who have fibromyalgia. There is so much of one's usual normal life lost to the average patient that depression is the natural result. Most FMS patients feel a tremendous sense of loss. So much is not the same as it was. Your role in a normal family is gone. You can't do many of the normal activities that you love to do. Your loss of energy further cuts down on life as you had known it before. All of these things lead rapidly to sadness and then to depression.

Researchers tell us that from 25 to 35 percent of all who have FMS also develop clinical depression. Some describe depression as a way of protecting the person by closing down much of his life to prevent any further trauma and stress.

This is often a period when the person's mind can try to come to grips with what he or she has already lost, and wonder about how to cope with that loss and how it is possible to move forward. The more lost life the person has suffered, the longer will be the depression.

Sleep patterns are usually impacted by depression. The lack of sleep causes more FMS problems, further deepening the depression and the endless cycle repeats itself to the detriment of the patient.

Most doctors say that depression should be treated if it lasts for more than six weeks.

Sometimes, even today, FMS patients are misdiagnosed by doctors who are well-intentioned but haven't the slightest idea what fibromyalgia is or how to treat it. The patient may be told—or the implication may be made—that she is making up the whole thing or that what she really needs is psychiatric help. This in itself can worsen the depression.

Make sure you understand the difference between depression and stress. Once the difference is recognized, treatment for both problems can be undertaken. No, they are not the same treatments.

Stress will surely help bring on depression and this in the long run may cause more stress. Depression is a state of being where you are continually sad, discouraged, feeling as if the whole world is against you and there simply is no reason to try to feel better.

When many fibromyalgia patients are correctly diagnosed, they already are in a state of depression at the same time. No one knows which comes first. We do know that FMS can produce depression. We're not quite sure if depression can produce the symptoms of FMS or not.

Here are some of the tests and common signals of depression:

- Not interested in usual activities.
- Experience continuing fatigue.
- Sleep patterns are distorted out of normal.
- A rapid gain or loss of more than 5 percent of body weight. (A 140 pound woman should not lose or gain more than seven pounds.)
- Serious mood swings.
- Thoughts of suicide or dying.
- Feelings of terrible guilt or of being worthless.
- Inability to think straight.
- Excessive irritability.
- Highly agitated.
- Avoiding best friends.

- Staying home all the time.
- Extreme problem concentrating.
- Lack of interest in sex.
- Problem anxiety.
- Headaches not from other problems.
- Constant lack of energy.
- A restless, slowed-down feeling.
- Hard time making decisions.
- Serious lack of deep sleep.
- Digestive problems.
- Fear of being alone.
- Nightmares about pain, loss or death.

Just trying to live with the constant pain and fatigue of FMS—along with a lack of good sleep—can easily push someone into a depression. Some of these symptoms may come one day, others the next day. Often there is crying for no reason, and a feeling of absolute loss of self-worth.

Don't confuse the occasional "bad day" or "down in the dumps" that normal people often have. To be a depression, the symptoms should show on a daily basis for two or three weeks. Then is the time to do something about them. The best way is to tell yourself, or convince a depressed friend, that some kind of professional help is needed.

DEPRESSION COMPLICATES FMS TREATMENT

One of the problems with depression is that it will mean that you probably will need to make some changes in your regular treatment of your FMS.

Talk it over with your doctor. He will have some medications to use to work on your depression and at the same time may want to increase or decrease some of your other medications aimed at your FMS. One thing he'll probably suggest is that you increase your daily exercise routine. If you don't have one, now is a brilliant time to start one. Do walking as a start. It's easy, simple, you don't need a partner to play against, and you can do it inside a mall in the winter or right around your residential block almost any time.

PSYCHOLOGICAL ROOT?

Some researchers say that they believe that depression is caused by some recognizable psychological defect in the patient.

Depression is found in a higher percentage of FMS patients than in the general public. Another study showed that there was a higher percentage of depression in immediate family members of FMS patients than there was in similar groups around someone with arthritis.

Later studies have tended to discount these theories, however. Now many doctors think that depression in FMS patients and in those with serious arthritis has been caused by the prime illness and is not the cause of that illness.

Chronic pain and constant fatigue can be enough to drop a person into depression. These two alone can cut into your normal activities, which mean less exercise, more pain that leads to withdrawal—all of which can work to deepen your depression.

WHO IS AT HIGH RISK FOR DEPRESSION?

The population as a whole has a problem with depression, not just FMS patients. Psychologists and psychiatrists from around the country have come up with a list that shows who has an increased risk for developing depression. This is not just fibromyalgia patients, but the population in general.

If you:

- Are a woman.
- Have been depressed before.
- Have little or no family or social support.
- Have a medical problem.
- Are post partum.
- Have had a recent highly stressful experience.
- Have made suicide attempts.
- Had clinical depression before age of 40.
- Abuse drugs or alcohol.
- Had incomplete treatment for prior depression.

• Have a family member who has been depressed.

This is a general situation list. If you have one or more of these risk factors, it does not mean that you will become depressed. It also doesn't mean that if you don't have any of these situations listed that you won't become depressed sometime in the future.

Depression is highly subjective. Situations that will throw one person into a deep depression may not affect another person at all.

Anytime that you feel that you are becoming depressed—and it's more than just a blue week—don't take chances: see your doctor and have a talk.

FIBROMYALGIA CAN LEAD TO DEPRESSION

We've said it before, but it bears repeating. Just the fact that you have fibromyalgia can result in your depression. This varies with case to case. Some people can resist the FMS symptoms, fight them, batter them down and go on living a more normal life. Others are crushed by the pain, the fatigue, the anxiety—and the result for them is a depression that tends to make their other symptoms worse.

Just discovering that you have FMS can be a shock that could be one of the factors in piling depression on top of the other fibromyalgia symptoms of aches and pains and hurts all over the place. The best bet here is to get that depression treated as quickly as you can by a doctor you know and trust, and kick one of the symptoms right out the window.

When you have FMS it's easy to start feeling sorry for yourself. Poor you. "Why did this have to happen to me?" These are fertile grounds for plain old negative thinking. Pretty soon you're negative not only about your sickness, but also about every aspect of your life. This is hard on family and friends, and can be fatal job-wise when you go to work.

This negative thinking can also lead you straight into the pit of depression. Then you'll really have something to cry about. As a preventive to depression, give some of these ideas a try to brighten your spirits, to simply make you feel better, to batter down the discouragement and frustrations. Remember "Happy Talk" from South Pacific? Dig it out and play it. Also try these:

- Turn on some favorite music.
- Take a friend out for coffee.
- Read a book out in the sunshine.
- Wear your favorite perfume when you are just at home.
- Make a list of your dream vacations.
- Luxuriate in a warm bubble bath.
- Go out for a massage.
- Watch a funny movie.
- Call a friend for a long talk.
- Go out to eat dinner.
- Have an expensive facial.

HIGH COST OF DEPRESSION

MIT has reported that depression is robbing American business of more than $44 billion a year—in lost time, in poor work, in missed meetings, people-caused accidents, and lower production.

Think what your own depression will cost you in lost wages, lost confidence of your supervisor, lost enjoyment of your family and friends because of your depression.

TREATING YOUR DEPRESSION

Depression comes in various levels of intensity from minor and low-level to the totally debilitating and dangerous forms. Most of the depression cases associated with FMS range from low to medium level. This can make it hard to detect, or for the patient even to realize that she is depressed.

If you or a friend think you might be depressed, that you are showing some of the traditional symptoms of depression mentioned above, it's time to talk to your doctor. She may make some suggestions and offer some medication, or she may send you scooting over to a psychologist or a physiciatrist.

Here is where a support group and your loyal friends might come into play. For low-level depression, often the support group can hold you up, offer some suggestions that they have used for the same problem and gradually help you work out of the small problems of depression that you were experiencing. The support group will be the best here, because if the group is of any size, it should contain one or more persons who have had the same symptoms you are having, and can tell you what they did and how it helped them kick the problem.

Your doctor may suggest a prescription drug. We'll get into that aspect of the treatment later in this chapter.

If a psychologist is suggested, be totally candid and open with him or her. Tell the doctor your personal history, your problems with FMS and how that affects you, and tell him/her what medications you are taking for the FMS. Then it's your job to follow the psychologist's directions to the letter.

EXERCISE CAN HELP

If you skipped the chapter on exercise, go back and read it. The fact is that exercise can help you manage your FMS symptoms, make you feel better generally, and do a lot of good for you just to be out and about. The second aspect of exercise is that it can help to relieve that low-level depression that you have. How? Nobody is exactly sure.

Exercise does boost the serotonin level in the brain. We know that this helps several aspects of FMS. The very fact that it is helping you to cope with and perhaps even reduce the devastating effects of some of the pain and fatigue and frustration might just be a big part of helping you kick your depression at the same time.

Remember with exercise every little bit helps. If you haven't been doing any, start out slow. Maybe get a friend and go to a closed mall. Winter or summer, morning, afternoon or evening, you can take a walk in nearly total safety— where it is warm or cool depending on the season, and where you can fool yourself that you're just taking a walk around and window shopping, when actually you are getting in a two mile walk. The idea is to start easy with exercising, and usually the easiest to do and get started with, is walking. Don't forget. If you haven't been exercising, and a low-level depression has you grumpy, give exercising a try.

One more benefit from a gentle, easy aerobic exercise such as walking. It will help you to decrease fluid retention in your body. Hey, you should be able to drop four or five pounds of fluid after a week or two of those daily, easy-to-do exercise routines.

WHAT YOU EAT CAN HELP

Yes, your diet can have an effect on your depression. The connection isn't A to B to C. Nothing so cut and dried. However it has been shown that an increase in serotonin can help you fight your depression. Exercise helps here as we saw above. What food you eat as well can be helpful.

This will have to be on a trial and error basis. Below is a list of foods that help boost your serotonin level. Try two at a time and see if they make any difference in how you feel. When you find the ones that help, try to get them into your diet at least once a day. You might want to go to the five small meals a day to keep an even level in your blood sugar and your energy quotient.

The list includes sherbet, bagels, bread, potatoes, cereal, rice, pasta, muffins, turkey and crackers.

So, give it a try. These foods may boost your serotonin level, help reduce your FMS symptoms, and at the same time reduce your depression level.

LIGHTS, ACTION

Ever heard of SAD? That's Seasonal Affective Disorder. It's what people have when, in the winter in less daylight time, they actually get depressed and sluggish and don't want to work. They can't work.

Psychologists recognize the disorder now and find they can reduce or end it with light treatments. There are specially made light booths where people are exposed to bright lights for given periods of time. The idea is that with the exposure to more than normal seasonal light, the body reacts as it would in the summer, and produces more serotonin. There is that word again.

Now doctors are experimenting with the idea that exposure

of FMS patients to these light booths should also produce more serotonin, which can be a help in reducing your depression.

Experiments have shown that some FMS patients have noticed a marked improvement in their mild depression after a thirty-minute exposure in this light booth. Others have needed up to two hours to get the same kind of relief.

Depressed? Turn on all the lights in the room and bathe yourself in a few two hundred-watt bulbs. It just might help.

PRESCRIPTION MEDICATIONS FOR DEPRESSION

Yes, if your doctor thinks that drugs are needed to help treat your depression, there are some on the shelf. Your medical advisor will make certain that you have tried the other non-drug treatments that we have covered above before he sends you to the pharmacy.

Tricyclics and tetracyclics are two drugs often used for several stages of depression. These work on reducing depression, and at the same time help the patient to get more stage 4 (deep) sleep. Such a deep sleep lets the body produce more serotonin for the central nervous system, which helps reduce many of the symptoms of FMS.

Amitriptyline is one of the drugs used to treat depression. It is an old medication and low-priced. Doctors find that it works well in about a third of their depressed patients. There are several drugs for depression and you and your doctor will want to experiment to see which one works best for you.

Your doctor will know which medications work against depression. Here are a few of the more commonly used antidepressant medications:

Norpramin, Effexor, Ascendin, Paxil, Remeron, Zoloft, Prozac, Serzone, Tofranil, Wellbutrin, Sinequan, and Surmontil.

Narcotic medications are generally not used for the treatment of depression. They can quickly become habit-forming and in many cases will aggravate depression and not help it. Then too, narcotic medications usually cause serious constipation if they are taken regularly.

Xanax—alprazolam—is often prescribed for anxiety. It can also be used to counter depression. Sometimes it is taken together with ibuprofen, and usually six to eight weeks are needed to see positive results.

CHAPTER 13

GOOD NUTRITION IS ESSENTIAL

No food that you eat or drink is going to cure your fibromyalgia. Most specialists in this field agree on that. However researchers are constantly on the hunt for a nutrition regimen that will help your body fight off diseases and hopefully prevent you from getting sick.

First comes eating healthy foods, and maintaining a reasonable weight for your body style. With these two basics, we can move on to more specifics. By healthy foods, we mean those that are low in fat and loaded with immunity boosting antioxidants and phytochemicals that work together to give you lots of energy—and perhaps minimize your fatigue, sleeplessness and muscle pain.

Keeping yourself in good health is a major project in itself. When you have the various problems of fibromyalgia weighing down the scales against you, the task becomes even more difficult and at the same time tremendously important.

A well-balanced diet of the food groups and with lots of fruit and vegetables and lots of water during the day can give you a leg up on the good nutrition factor. Naturally good health is the total of at least three factors: a sound, workable body; a clear and active mind, and a bundle of emotions that are controlled and practical.

Those with FMS have a host of problems, and poor nutrition should not be added to the list of woes. The facts are that proper nutrition and mind/emotional health can actually help to reduce the severity of most of the symptoms of fibromyalgia. It's one area where you can do something that just might help your pains and fatigue.

Your body is not a simple machine. All your car needs is some gas and oil and it runs for a hundred thousand miles. Your body must have a variety of elements to function correctly. These include protein, fats, carbohydrates, fiber, vitamins, phytochemicals and minerals.

A recent study showed that your body needs 60 different minerals every day to survive—along with 16 vitamins, 90 nutrients, 3 essential fatty acids, and 12 essential amino acids. Nutritionists tell us not to worry, a balanced diet will provide all of these elements and even more. But not all of us bother to eat a healthy diet. Some folks don't like collard greens, broccoli or spinach. The truth is, all of us have to work at getting a healthy diet every day. We're going to show you how before long.

Some people say that foods which are organically grown have more healthful elements in them of vitamins, acids and nutrients. Don't bank on it. Experts disagree on just how much better true organic-grown fruits and vegetables are. Then there is the problem of the truthfulness of the "organically grown" label on many of the items now in stores. Who checks to be sure those carrots came from a true organic farm?

ONE WAY YOU HAVE SOME CONTROL

A lot of the aches and pains and problems brought on by fibromyalgia you have no control over. But when it comes to wellness eating you do have complete control. It starts with shopping and ends up on your table. Just knowing that you are eating a balanced diet and getting your vitamins can have a beneficial effect far beyond the calories and vitamins. It gives you a psychological boost knowing that you're doing something to help fight your disease.

ANTIOXIDANTS

You've heard of these. They are the cure. The problem they fight is cells in your body on the warpath. These are called free radicals and they have one electron missing for some unhealthy reason. They go charging around your body attacking anything they can and are thought to be one of the underlying causes of a host of diseases from cancer to fibromyalgia. How to fight them?

Antioxidants are the answer. They are essential nutrients that help protect your body and at the same time attack the free cells and stabilize them so they can't harm your body.

They act to protect healthy cells. So where do you get a lot of these antioxidants? From foods that are rich in beta-carotene and vitamins E and C. Some researchers say that these antioxidants can help with some types of arthritis and give your whole immune system a big boost. This also means they probably help with your pains, your fatigue and even your sleep disruption.

WHERE TO GET ANTIOXIDANTS

Number one source is good old beta-carotene. It's all over the place. Think of carrots, cantaloupe, apricots, spinach, and pumpkins. The beta-carotene is converted to vitamin A in the body and it is assimilated.

Other sources of beta-carotene are: broccoli, collard greens, kale, peaches, red peppers, sweet potatoes, papayas, winter squash, turnip greens and tomatoes.

VITAMIN E IS ESSENTIAL

Getting enough vitamin E is also essential in a healthy diet to help combat your fibromyalgia. Vitamin E helps to keep the membranes of your body's cells healthy. Vitamin E also has an antioxidant effect and that helps your general health as well. Vitamin E is also good for your heart, helping to lower the risk of a heart attack or coronary heart disease.

The food you eat furnishes vitamin E mainly through veg-etables, seed oils, margarine, nuts, wheat germ and vegetable oils. Which means you probably don't get enough. Supplements abound in E and are available at any food or drug store. Look for the 200 or 400 IU tablets.

GOOD OLD VITAMIN C

Another building block of a good nutritional menu includes Vitamin C, also called ascorbic acid. This basically helps a scratch or a wound to heal faster and generally protects us against infection. If your body is seriously wounded or ill, or under stress, the level of ascorbic acid is usually low in your bloodstream. It is also depressed in older people, so think about a supplement here, some 500 IUs daily.

Vitamin C also helps you to be more alert and increases your ability to concentrate because it produces the brain chemical norepinephrine. Another reason to be sure that you get enough Vitamin C. Where from?

Eat lots of these: strawberries, tomatoes, peppers, broccoli, oranges, potatoes, kiwi, cantaloupes, and grapefruit juice.

WHAT ARE PHYTOCHEMICALS?

They are nutrient and non-nutrient compounds found in plant-based foods. Research by nutrition experts say that a wide variety of foods in your diet can do more than just provide good nutrient intake. These foods can also provide these phytochemicals that are thought to be vital in protection against many diseases.

These phytochemicals are a part of all plants—including food plants. If you set up your plate with a variety of fruits and vegetables along with the other elements of a good diet, you should be getting enough of these vital chemicals.

Which foods have the most phytochemicals?

- Carrots
- Apricots
- Sweet potatoes
- Cabbage
- Broccoli
- Cauliflower

- Soybeans
- Tomatoes
- Red peppers
- Onions
- Brussels sprouts

Here are six ways to add phytochemicals to your menu:

1. Add chopped up fruit to your muffins, yogurt, ice cream, and cereal.
2. Have twice-a-day snacks of cut up broccoli, cauliflower, carrots and peppers. A dip works great here.
3. Put spinach, sliced carrots and raw broccoli along with shredded cabbage in your vegetable salads.
4. Feature steamed cabbage, Brussels sprouts or broccoli in your daily menus.
5. Keep natural herbs available in your garden for picking; also stock ginger, garlic, chives and parsley for ready use.
6. Tomato salsa mixed with nonfat yogurt makes a good cracker dip.

PUNCHING UP YOUR IMMUNE SYSTEM

Your immune system is that nearly automatic device in your body that fights off diseases, viruses, infections and other bad guys that get into your body. There are ways to help your immune system to remain healthy and active, so your body can remain healthy and active, and so it can help you fight your pains and problems from fibromyalgia.

The last thing you want is to come down with a month-long cold or a bout with the flu or some other health problem. You don't want two big sicknesses on top of each other. You need to do everything you can to keep yourself well: have your flu shot, wash your hands frequently if you make a lot of social contacts, and take care of your general health. You also want to boost your immune system to grab those germs that you often can't help but host.

GET HELP FROM BIOFLAVINOIDS

What are they? Flavinoids is a term for over four thousand compounds that give colors to fruits and vegetables. One big source of flavinoids for you is the soft and white inner skin on all citrus fruits. Usually we peel those white things off and throw them away. Not the next time. They can help you. They include key nutrients that can give your natural immune system a boost.

There are a lot of these biochemicals with Vitamin C in plants and they can also act as antioxidants. Where to look to get more of these flavinoids in your diet? For sure in grapefruit, lemons, limes and oranges. Also give a bite to cherries, black currants, plums, apricots, grapes, blackberries and papaya.

For flavinoids from vegetables, eat broccoli, green peppers, squash, tomatoes, eggplant and parsley.

Another compound that can help your immune system— and in the process may deter or decrease the severity of your FMS symptoms—includes quercetin. This highly concentrated type of bioflavinoid is obtained through eating citrus fruits, broccoli, yellow and red onions. Hesperidin is another bioflavinoid from citrus. This one is reported to raise your blood level, thereby getting more nutrients and oxygen to your muscles and organs for better overall health.

Glutathione is another bioflavinoid compound, this one found in watermelon, that can help to strengthen your immune system so it can fight your body's problems. This compound is also found in cruciferous vegetables, or the mustard family of plants.

THREE SQUARE MEALS A DAY?

In spite of what you may have heard, three big meals a day are not the best way to eat for healthy living. Especially if you have fibromyalgia. What is better? The nutritional experts tell us that five lighter meals a day are better for a person. This is doubly true for FMS patients.

Five smaller meals spaced out through the day lets the body have a more continuous supply of nutrients and maintains the energy level better than the feast and famine three-meal regimen.

Yes, these non-traditional food intakes can be in the form of snacks—healthy ones such as fruit juices, mixed fruit, nuts and berries. Here are some general suggestions for healthy eating for fibromyalgia patients.

Metabolism is the key here. By eating every three hours or so during the day—and keeping them healthy type meals and snacks— you'll keep your metabolism up, and not have those hungry, low energy times. Yes, it works.

For those between meal snacks, be sure you pick the healthy ones: an apple, a banana, almost any fruit, and whole grain crackers, or a nice orange or carrot. Keep the snacks simple to prepare and to carry, as well as to eat. Stay away from candy bars, milkshakes, cookies and sugar coated cereals.

You may wish to prepare and leave nutritious snacks at work and around the house. Some more good snacks include nuts, pretzels and popcorn. If you have a microwave at the office, use the unbuttered type popcorn. Do you have enough popcorn to share?

Remember complex carbohydrates when you buy your groceries and for meals. They should make up 70 percent of your calories for the day. The carbos provide the raw material your body burns to keep itself moving and working and for healing any small muscle tears. This is doubly important for FMS patients since one of the main problems is with your muscles and connective tissue.

These complex carbos, especially when eaten on a five-meal-a-day plan, help keep your energy level high, and fight the fatigue that often plagues you.

Nutritionists say there are 90 nutrients the body needs every day. You don't even have to know what they are, just concentrate on eating a wide variety of foods including a lot of fresh fruit and vegetables. These provide you with your carbos, proteins and vitamins and minerals you need for a healthy life.

This also means you'll have the best chance to fight your FMS and get better.

As a fibromyalgia patient, you should eliminate red meat from your diet. Many experts say it is detrimental to FMS patients. Get your protein instead from beans, nuts, vegetables, chicken, turkey, tuna and other fish. Here you need not more than 15% of your diet in protein.

Fat is always a problem. It should make up about 20 percent of your diet. Fat has taken a beating lately. Most of us eat too much fat, and fat of the bad kind. You need some fat for a healthy life. Watch the labels on foods and try for the monounsaturated and polyunsaturated fats in such foods as olive, safflower, canola, peanut and corn oils.

Do you need purified or bottled water in your diet? Most nutritionists say it would be fine, but really not needed. In almost all of the water districts in the nation, the water is not detrimental to your health. If you're a strong believer in drinking and using distilled or purified water only, it can't hurt.

Go easy on fast food. A hamburger and fries won't kill you, but don't eat out that way every day. Concentrate more on fresh vegetables and fruits and chicken and turkey and the good things mentioned above.

As an FMS patient, you should not be drinking coffee or colas. Avoiding caffeine will make a difference. Some patients report immediate results with lowered anxiety and nervousness. Did you know that champion rifle marksmen never drink coffee during or for several hours before a match? The caffeine makes them jumpy enough to make a difference in their final scores.

KEEP FIBER IN YOUR DIET

Yes, almost all of us should put more fiber into our diet. Fiber is that part of fruits and vegetables that won't digest—little sticks that are pushed through your digestive tract, keeping the whole bunch moving and not allowing the harmful elements to stay in your system long enough to let cancer causing agents act.

Fiber is one big advantage you get when you eat five or more servings of vegetables every day. Your high fiber diet cuts the risk of cancers of the colon by 70 percent. It also lowers your risk for developing gallstones and kidney stones and helps tremendously with regular bowel movements.

If it has time, fiber will ferment in the colon, increasing the amount of oxygen, which reduces the action of harmful bacteria.

Another reason for your five servings of fruits and vegetables every day. Use these fruits and veggies without peeling them. Wash carefully and then chomp away. Other high fiber foods include figs, dried beans, prunes, peas and oats—as in oatmeal, oat cereal and even oat cookies. Do they count? Not sure, but even more fiber comes to you through wheat bran and those seven grain breads and other whole grain foods— pasta, rice and whole grain cereals.

More high fiber foods: acorn squash, baked potatoes, blueberries lentils, pumpkins, raspberries, sweet potatoes and strawberries.

VITAMINS, MINERALS AND ENZYMES

We've touched lightly on some of these before: now let's take a more detailed look at them and bunch them all together. These are weapons you can use to make your body healthier and at the same time help you fight against fibromyalgia. Let's take a look:

VITAMIN C: You know that citrus fruits are the best source of vitamin C. It is one of the champion antioxidants on the market, and that's good. Also high in C are strawberries, bananas, papayas, mangos, raspberries, tomatoes, cantaloupe, and pineapples.

Vegetables get equal time here for vitamin C production including broccoli, Brussels sprouts, cabbage, asparagus, collard greens, red peppers and potatoes.

The best way to go for your veggies is to cook them quickly, as raw as you can take them. Heat can destroy the goodness in those veggies and they come out about as nutritious as cardboard. Your best bet for the fruits is to eat them raw and leave the skin on when possible. Actually, banana skins are not all that tasty.

BETA-CAROTENE: this is the best known of all the dozens of carotinoids, and brings you vitamin A through the plant world.

Many people forget that dark and green leafy vegetables are a good source of beta carotene. These include broccoli, spinach, kale, parsley, collard greens, dandelion greens and others.

The top source of beta-carotene comes from carrots, sweet potatoes, mangos, papayas, melons, pumpkins, cantaloupe, and apricots. If it's yellow or orange, it's probably a good source of Vitamin A.

VITAMIN E: Another anti-oxidant, vitamin E can be found primarily in safflower oil, nuts, sunflower seeds, wheat germ, avocados, dried prunes, whole grain cereals and breads, asparagus, and broccoli.

MANGANESE: The pituitary gland relies on trace elements of manganese for proper functioning. This mineral also helps the healthy operation of the rest of the body's glands. It is important to FMS patients because it helps the body to use glucose, which produces energy and at the same time helps the central nervous system to stay on track.

SELENIUM: Many researchers believe that selenium helps accelerate your immune system by protecting your cells from the toxic effect of free radicals. Foods are a good source of natural selenium, including wheat breads, salmon, tuna, shrimp and sunflower seeds.

CHROMIUM PICOLINATE: Another trace mineral important to help the body use fatty acids and in the metabolism of glucose to produce energy. It also helps the body to utilize insulin more efficiently. Not readily available in foods, it is available in tablet form in health food stores.

MALIC ACID: Works in the production of bodily energy. It is also important in reducing the bad effects of aluminum in your body.

Put it in tandem with magnesium and they are effective in

helping to heal some of the problems of fibromyalgia. A health food store item.

Magnesium: Is part of the enzyme system in the body. Can be greatly important in healing fibromyalgia tissue problems. Most FMS patients are lacking in normal magnesium levels. It also helps to absorb calcium, phosphorus, potassium, all the B vitamins, and vitamins E and C. With malic acid it helps with energy production for the body.

Zinc: Another trace mineral that helps your body absorb vitamins, helps grow skin, nails and hair, and is a part of digestion and metabolism. An important one. It works in your body only in association with vitamin A. You can ingest zinc though the herb licorice, ginseng and chalk. Also a health food store item in tablet form.

Boron: A trace mineral that you can find in cauliflower and apples. Boron is an antioxidant and is vital to maintaining healthy muscles. This means it helps keep the cells from releasing free radicals that the body must track down and zap.

Rice Bran Extract: You may never have heard of this one. This extract is said to be 6,000 times stronger than vitamin E. Why don't we just take this one and forget vitamin E? No one will tell us.

Glucosamine: Has been shown to be important in reducing sensitivity and pain in soft tissue areas of FMS patients. It also is effective for the improvement of arthritis. It is described as being a substance that determines how many water-holding molecules can be retained in cartilage.

Coenzyme Q-10: This is an enzyme that is a vital part of the immune system. For a fibromyalgia patient, it can increase circulation and boost your energy level.

Proanthocyanidins: This comes from pycnogenol, which comes from grape seed extract and is a strong antioxidant. It is reported to be highly efficient in boosting the immune system and a good treatment for fibromyalgia patients.

As mentioned before, not all of these minerals and enzymes mentioned above can be obtained by eating the right diet. Some of them must come in the form of food supplements from your neighborhood health food store.

Check with your doctor to go over your diet and then decide which of the supplements will help you to achieve better recovery and a better life style. Most doctors agree that with today's use of chemicals and pesticides in our agriculture, it is tough to get enough vital vitamins, minerals and enzymes by diet alone. When it comes to food supplements, the lowest price isn't always the best buy—read the labels.

SOME HEALTHY EATING FOODS

There are all sorts of diets and food lists and dos and don'ts about eating healthy. Here are some foods that, when all the dust settles, come out on most nutritionists' lists of healthy foods. Take a look, give them a try.

Say you don't like one of them, say spinach? Tough, learn to eat it, or dig into the nutrition and get other foods that will do the same thing it does. Check out this bunch.

DAIRY FOODS

Dairy products are low priced, available and a staple in most American diets today. Cheeses, cottage cheese, skimmed milk, buttermilk, no-fat milk, yogurt and ice cream are all good ways to provide top nutrients to your body for finely tuned operation. The vitamin D and calcium in milk products help maintain strong bones and ward off broken bones. For older people, milk is a good way to help prevent osteoporosis. Low-fat milk products can help you keep your blood pressure down as well.

WHAT ABOUT GREEN TEA?

Researchers now say that green tea may be a factor in preventing strokes and cardiovascular problems. Green tea also contains a high level antioxidant that does a lot of good things for the whole body. Research continues here but early reports offer the possibility that green tea may help reduce the chances of developing osteoporosis as well as these cancers: lung, skin, esophageal, pancreatic and breast. One of the chemicals in green tea fights against an enzyme in cancer growth.

Home free? Not quite. If you are on a no-caffeine pro-gram, the sad fact here is that one cup of green tea steeped for three minutes has from 20 to 50 mg of caffeine. A cup of cof-fee has up to 125 mg of caffeine.

GOOD OLD BROCCOLI

You've seen broccoli mentioned many times in this healthy eating food section. Broccoli is full of all sorts of phytochemi-cals that contain a number of top dietary nutrition and healing powers. Remember: don't cook it to death. Steaming is best and raw is better. If you want to stock up on those cancer fighting phytochemicals in your daily diet, find broccoli sprouts at specialty food stores. These sprouts contain 100 times as many of one of the cancer fighting chemicals as regu-lar broccoli. And they are green.

SPINACH

Folic acid is one of the nutrients that does a lot for your body, including fighting clogged arteries. The villain is homo-cysteine: a blood protein that helps clogging. It is a by-product of a high protein diet. To counteract this, eat lots of spinach and other dark green vegetables, citrus fruits and juices, enriched breads and whole grains. Spinach also has lots of vita-mins C and A, beta-carotene and potassium—all extremely important to your good health. Good old spinach is also important in fighting macular degeneration, one of the leading causes of near-blindness in older people.

OLIVE OIL

You don't have to be Italian to like olive oil. It should be the cooking oil of choice for every kitchen. Olive oil is one of the mono-unsaturated fats that is more healthy for you than the other vegetable cooking oils and margarine. Proof? Olive oil is used almost exclusively in Mediterranean countries, and in those areas breast cancer is 50% lower than it is in the United States. The olive oil use is said to be the majority of the reason for lower breast cancer there.

FISHY TALE

This is swinging a little away from fibromyalgia, but it does have a bearing. If you drop dead suddenly from cardiac arrest, all the fibromyalgia help in the world will be useless. So bear with this section on your general health. Eating fish once or twice a week can cut down on the risk of a sudden heart attack. In one large-scale study, the researchers found that men who ate fish once a week had half the risk of sudden cardiac death as men in the study who had fish once a month or less. N-3 fatty acid is the good guy here. It's in fish, and has some as yet undetermined effect on the body. It helps, so have another helping of fish. All seafood is good for you, but these are especially helpful: whitefish, scallops, sardines, tuna, salmon, lobster, anchovies, bluefish and mackerel.

RED GRAPES

Activin is a new super antioxidant recently discovered that is contained in the seeds of red grapes. Researchers are working on it, but they believe that the seeds themselves, or things made from red grapes such as red wine, grape juice, or the grapes themselves, are powerful. They may give real protection against rheumatoid arthritis, heart disease and cancer. Many believe that activin is seven times more powerful than the antioxidants in vitamins E and C and in beta-carotene. Yes, it looks like red wine is more healthful for you than white wine.

OH BOY...SOY!

We have known for twenty years that soy protein, which comes from soybeans, is a cheap and healthy substitute for meat. Soy products don't have any saturated fat. Those who are allergic to dairy foods can eat soy with no problems. Asians eat a lot of soy foods, and they have much lower incidence of breast and prostate cancer, heart disease and osteoporosis than Americans do. Americans who eat some type of soy food once or more a week have half the risk of developing polyps that can lead to cancer as those who don't eat any soy. You hate tofu? Fine, don't use it. There are other types of soy products on the market now, including fortified soymilk, textured vegetable protein, tahini, and soy nuts. Hey, the stuff is good for you.

GARLIC

Garlic has two or three benefits for you besides the taste it gives otherwise tasteless food. Garlic has in it chemicals just like a prescription drug given to lower blood pressure. Pills of garlic can lower your blood pressure by dilating blood vessels so they simply hold more blood and reduce the pressure. New research shows that garlic and onions can stop the growth of nitrosamines. These are dangerous carcinogens that may produce cancers in the breasts, colon and liver.

TOMATOES

Yes, a healthy food that almost everyone likes. Tomatoes have proven to contain a powerful antioxidant called lycopene. Researchers say it is much more potent than beta-carotene, vitamin E, or alpha-carotene. Lycopene gives you protection against several cancers and heart disease. You get more useable lycopene from tomatoes when they are cooked, rather than raw. The cooking sets up the lycopene so it can be assimilated by the body.

FAT GRAMS AND CALORIES DO COUNT

Now, with all of the above food items to consider, you will also want to be careful about how much fat and how many calories that you eat. Don't overeat. It's too easy to do these days. Most of us simply eat too much.

For a quick look at how many fat grams and calories certain foods have, please turn to the back of the book to Appendix A.

There is no final word about food and general health and your fibromyalgia. The best advice is to watch your diet so you will be eating in such a way that it will bring you the best health possible. This better health should give you a chance at swifter healing of your fibromyalgia aches, pains and problems. At the least, better nutrition will mean more energy for you, and should also give your immune system a boost. That could mean more inside healing by your body, and good news for you.

CHAPTER 14

MINERALS, VITAMINS AND HERBAL REMEDIES

Many of the medicines we use every day came originally from tree bark or leaves or some other plant or natural growth. These have worked into our medical world and are now taken for granted. Today there are hundreds of other herbs and natural supplements out there that specialists in those fields say can be of tremendous help to the general public if only we would try them.

Usually doctors don't have time to know about these fields. They have a tough time just keeping up with the latest in medicines and new remedies in their medical fields. Many of these same physicians will also suggest that some of the products now available may be able to help those with fibromyalgia.

The secret here is to find out just which ones may help. Consult with a herbologist or a naturopath, or someone who understands about herbs and other supplements and determine which might be best for you.

When you do get a recommendation, talk it over with your doctor. She may know of some of the substances that could harm more than help FMS. Generally it's not good planning to self-treat with herbs and supplements without the advice of your doctor.

MINERALS

Medical science has done and continues to do great volumes of research into minerals and the part they play in the body. Minerals in minute amounts are absolutely vital to your good health. Most of these trace elements of minerals can't be stored in the body, and must be ingested on a daily basis. Don't panic. Most of these trace minerals come to you naturally through the food that you eat. If you are eating anywhere near a healthy diet, you're probably getting enough of these minerals.

Without these minerals, the vitamins, amino acids, enzymes, fats and carbohydrates can't be absorbed by the body to perform their necessary functions. You also need minerals to improve your brain function and mental agility, to normalize your heartbeat, keep your nervous system on track, increase your energy, fight fatigue, and assist in the metabolic process.

There are 17 trace elements of minerals that are essential to your body's functioning.

Some health food experts say that many people don't get enough trace minerals because these minerals are vanishing from our food supply due to food processing, the way foods are grown and the time from field to table.

For some, adding these minerals to the diet becomes an important element of their existence.

Here are some of the minerals that are vital to fibromyalgia patients:

MAGNESIUM: Most experts say that magnesium is an anti-stress mineral. It is a major controller of cellular activity, and helps your DNA and RNA to function correctly. Magnesium can calm you down and, when taken before bedtime, can help you settle down and even help you get to sleep. Magnesium is one of those trace elements that can't be stored and must be ingested daily in food or in pill form.

You might run short on magnesium in your system during times of stress, diarrhea, diabetes or kidney problems. You might also be deficient in magnesium if you are depressed, notice muscle weakness, irritability, nausea, muscle cramps and insomnia.

CALCIUM: Calcium is the most abundant mineral in the human body. That makes it absolutely essential to good health. Most of the calcium in your body is located in your bones and your teeth. It also helps in the transmission of nerve signals, muscular movement of the intestines, and the normal and smooth functioning of the heart muscles. A calcium supplement is another one that can have a calming effect on a person when taken before bedtime. This helps to relax your muscles. Calcium deficiency may result in leg numbness, tingling of the feet, fingers and lips, sensitivity to noise and even muscle cramps.

CHROMIUM: We need chromium in our system to help synthesize fatty acids and to metabolize blood sugars to produce energy. It can also increase the efficiency of insulin. You might be deficient in chromium if you have a sudden weight loss, can't tolerate glucose and have bouts with mental confusion.

POTASSIUM: Potassium is vital to your health. It maintains normal heart and muscle functioning, keeps nerve impulses moving, and promotes normal growth in children. Potassium is also essential in stimulating nerve impulses, which cause muscle contractions. You may be short on potassium if you have weakness and soreness, muscle twitches, rapid or erratic heartbeat, fatigue, nervousness, high cholesterol, or insomnia.

ZINC: Trace elements of zinc in your system are the do-everything healer. It is vital for enzymes in the brain that repair cells. It is vital for your vision, taste and hearing, and helps to form your hair, nails and skin.

Zinc helps the body to absorb vitamins, and works with enzymes in digestion and metabolism. You could be short on zinc if you have an unusual memory loss, depression, diarrhea, brittle nails, hair loss or fatigue.

SELENIUM: Selenium is a potent antioxidant, and is needed to help the immune system to function. It helps the use of other nutrients including vitamin E. It helps cell membranes and with DNA metabolism. Selenium also helps protect the body from drug toxicity and heavy metals such as aluminum, cadmium and mercury.

PHOSPHORUS: Phosphorus works with calcium, and it too is found mainly in your teeth and bones. You can cut down on your phosphorus levels by drinking too many carbonated beverages, by a lack of vitamin D, and plain old stress. For fibromyalgia patients, phosphorus is essential since it aids in the oxidation of carbohydrates and at the same time helps produce energy. If you're low on phosphorus you may have a loss of appetite, a nervous disorder, insomnia or irregular breathing.

IODINE: Your body needs trace elements of iodine for your thyroid gland. With iodine your thyroid can regulate the body's energy production. If your thyroid doesn't work correctly, you'll be lethargic and suffer fatigue. Other problems with not enough iodine in your system include dry hair, cold hands and feet, swollen fingers and toes, and irritability.

VANADIUM: This trace mineral is not well researched yet, but experts think that it helps prevent heart disease. Vanadium is a co-factor to insulin and, with chromium, helps break down fats and sugars, which helps to keep coronary arteries clear. This trace mineral is also thought to be a factor in the creation of energy.

MANGANESE: Trace levels of manganese are found in nearly every part of your body. It is vital for the utilization of glucose. It is also important in the normal operation of your central nervous system, proper brain function, normal muscle use and for energy production. If you don't have enough manganese you could become suddenly hard of hearing, have nausea and dizziness, strained knees, and muscle coordination problems.

IRON: Most people know that both men and women need iron, yet not everyone gets enough iron in his or her diet. Your body absorbs iron easily but needs enough hydrochloric acid to utilize the iron. You also need enough vitamin C and E to get the most value from your iron intake. Iron is best known to help form hemoglobin. That's what they test you for at the blood bank before you give blood. Most women need more iron than men do.

WHAT ABOUT VITAMINS?

A lot of fibromyalgia patients suffer from vitamin deficiency and don't know it. Vitamins have been known and prescribed and self-administered for years. Most vitamins were discovered and identified between 1925 and 1930, but still many people ignore them. Most vitamins can be obtained through a good, well-rounded diet. However, millions of people take supplementary vitamins.

There are two classes of vitamins: water-soluble and fat-soluble. Most are the water type, and combine with water to work in the body. If they are not used they are discharged from the body through the urine. That means they are available for use for only a few hours before they are excreted. These vitamins, mainly the B and C complex ones, need to be ingested through food or pill form at least once a day.

Fat-soluble vitamins include A, D, K and E which combine with fats in the body, are absorbed by fats and stay available in the body for a much longer time.

For the best utilization, vitamins of both types should be taken before meals. You probably know about vitamins and what you need. Here is a quick look at them.

VITAMIN A: Vitamin A is a fat-soluble type, so too much of it can build up a toxicity in the system. Larger amounts of A can be obtained through taking large doses of beta-carotene which is not toxic and converts into vitamin A when it is needed. Amounts of up to 25,000 IU can be taken with no harmful effects. Vitamin A treats skin problems, fights infection, maintains and repairs muscle tissue, and aids in the health of bones, skin and teeth.

VITAMIN C: Vitamin C is also called ascorbic acid and is water-soluble. It helps prevent infection by destroying viruses and bacteria, promotes the activity of white blood cells, is a potent antioxidant and fights stress. Vitamin C also helps with the formation of collagen, is essential for good bones, teeth and skin, and aids the growth of children. It also helps the neurotransmitters in the brain and, when matched with bioflavinoids, assists the adrenal and immune functions.

VITAMIN E: This one is the best bet in the vitamin field to help fibromyalgia patients relax and calm down. Selenium increases the potency of Vitamin E. Vitamin E helps control unsaturated fats and may reduce cholesterol, keeps your brain functioning normally and protects several of your glands during bouts of stress. E is a strong antioxidant and is needed for blood clotting, maintaining muscles and nerves, and for lung metabolism.

VITAMIN B COMPLEX: B vitamins help calm a person and promote good mental health—two good reasons fibromyalgia patients need to take their B complex vitamins. They also are important in the production of serotonin, another calming chemical. When you're short on the B vitamins you may have trouble handling stress.

The B vitamins also help good brain function and to improve your concentration and memory.

VITAMIN B-1—THIAMIN: B-1 is vital for many body functions including digestion, muscle metabolism, blood cell metabolism, pain inhibition and to produce energy. Since it is water-soluble, it can be kept in the body for only a short time—six to eight hours. That's why you need to take more vitamin B-1 in food or as a supplement daily. Herbs that contain B-1 include peppermint, slippery elm, gotu kola and ginseng.

VITAMIN B-2—RIBOFLAVIN: You need B-2 for antibody formation, cell respiration, fat and carbohydrate metabolism, and red blood formation. B-2 is another water-soluble one, so it must be added to your diet daily. B-2 is essential for proper enzyme formation, tissue formation and normal children's growth. B-2 is found in the same herbs as B-1 plus kelp.

VITAMIN B-3—NIACINAMIDE: This one helps the body to produce insulin, male and female hormones and thyroxin, helps circulation, acid production, and histamine activation. Without enough B-3 you could develop hypoglycemia, memory loss, confusion, ringing in the ears and depression.

VITAMIN B-6—PYRIDOXINE: B-6 is the ticket for converting fats and proteins into energy. It also helps with the production of red blood cells, and the proper chemical balance of the body. Fibromyalgia patients who are suffering from stress will find B-6 especially helpful. But be careful. Too much B-6 can cause a folic acid deficiency.

VITAMIN B-12—COBALAMIN: Here B-12 is vital for fat, protein and carbohydrate metabolism, iron absorption, blood cell formation and to give your red blood cells a longer life. If you are a dedicated vegetarian, you'll need to supplement your diet with B-12. If you don't get enough B-12 you could have memory loss, headaches, dizziness, muscle weakness, fatigue, depression and paranoia.

BIOTIN: Biotin is needed if you are under extreme stress, or are experiencing nutrient malabsorption or have a poor nutrition program. Biotin aids in the metabolism of protein, fat and carbohydrates, in fatty acid production and cell growth.

PANTOTHENIC ACID: This particular acid is used in the normal functioning of muscle tissue and protects various membranes from being infected. It helps in energy conversion, blood stimulation and detoxification. If your fibromyalgia puts you under difficult stress, try some pantothenic acid for relief.

PARA AMINO BENZOIC ACID (PABA): PABA helps with protein metabolism and promotes growth and blood cell formation. A deficiency here can mean depression, fatigue constipation, nervousness and irritability.

VITAMIN P (BIOFLAVINOIDS): Bioflavinoids work in harness with Vitamin C to make stronger your connective tissue and capillaries. They are also important to help your body to utilize most of the other nutrients.

CAN HERBS HELP?

The bark, leaves, roots, fruits and flowers of various plants have been providing mankind down through the ages with certain healing agents. Today these herbal remedies are gaining more stature in the medical community. Indeed some of the herbal remedies of many years ago are now recognized medical compounds.

Herbs, as with any plant, contain various biochemical elements such as hormones, enzymes, vitamins, minerals, essential fatty acids, chlorophyll, fiber and many other properties. Herbs also contain vitamins, minerals and other nutrients the body needs.

These herbs need to be used only after consulting with a specialist, and usually they should not be used in conjunction with prescription medications unless monitored by a physician.

Single herbs do not always solve a problem. Usually they are prescribed in combinations.

Here is a list of herbs and nutrients that may be of some value to fibromyalgia patients.

VALERIAN: An herb used widely for nervous tension and anxiety. As a natural sedative it can improve sleep quality and help with insomnia as well as work to relieve depression. It is a safe non-narcotic herb used for heart palpitations, muscle spasms and arthritis. It is rich in calcium, magnesium and selenium as well as zinc and vitamins A and C.

CHAMOMILE: Chamomile promotes relaxation and sleep, aids digestion, and helps assimilate food. It is high in calcium and magnesium, which strengthens the nervous system. Helping here are vitamins A, C, F, and B complex. Selenium and zinc—important for the immune system—are also part of chamomile. It also contains tryptophan, to promote sleep.

PASSIONFLOWER: This herb is used in combination with other herbs to promote circulation and help with nervousness. Another combination works for insomnia and to combat nervous tension, anxiety, stress and restlessness.

RED CLOVER: Usually used in its liquid form, red clover is a blood purifier and blood builder, and helps produce energy to strengthen the immune system. It is high in vitamin A, and is often used in combination with other herbs. It is said to have antibiotic properties handy in fighting many diseases. It is good for fibromyalgia patients since it is high in selenium for good nutrition. Red clover also contains calcium and magnesium, sodium, copper and manganese.

GOLDENSEAL: This herb is said to boost the glandular system and at the same time promote hormone production. It also can help regulate liver function since it is said to be a natural insulin which provides the body with the nutrients needed to produce its own insulin. It has natural antibiotics to fight infection. This is due to its alkaloid nature which includes berberine.

ALOE VERA: This cactus-like plant is really from the lily family and is great for treating sunburn and radiation burns. For sunburn, it can be broken off a living plant and the juices spread over the burn. It relieves burning and stinging and helps heal.

When used internally, it can help move matter along the intestines, promote healing, and aid in digestion. This herb is high in selenium and vitamin C—two potent antioxidants. It also has vitamins A and B complex, phosphorus, magnesium, niacin, zinc and potassium.

GINSENG: This is one of the oldest herbs known to man. Some say also the most beneficial. It is said to help fight bronchitis and heart disease, reduce blood cholesterol, increase physical stamina, improve brain function and memory, and build the immune system. It is said to be the most potent of the herbs since it benefits the heart and circulation, prevents arteriosclerosis and normalizes blood pressure. It has so many good properties it must be valuable as well for those with fibromyalgia.

GOTU KOLA: This herb is billed as good for depression by fighting mental fatigue and memory loss. Some call it "brain food" since they say it energizes brain function. Gotu Kola is high in magnesium and vitamins A, C, B1, B2 and K. It also has manganese, niacin, calcium, zinc, and sodium.

SLIPPERY ELM: This powerful herb is great for fibromyalgia patients. It is a demulcent, buffering against irritations and inflammations of the mucous membrane. It also helps the adrenal gland and assists in both internal an external healing. It is a blood builder and helps the cardiovascular system. For vitamin and mineral content, it is about equal to that of oatmeal. The seven most important minerals are all contained in

Slippery Elm.

ROSEMARY: This common garden herb is best known as a replacement for aspirin to treat headaches. It also helps in fighting stress and improving memory. It is also high in calcium and said to be a top benefit to the whole nervous system.

ADDITIONAL VALUABLE SUPPLEMENTS

MELATONIN: Many authorities think that melatonin is a big help for those with sleep problems—a major problem for fibromyalgia patients. Melatonin is produced by a gland found in the middle of the brain, called the pineal gland. Generally the pineal gland releases melatonin if the eye is not receiving light. This means that melatonin can help control our sleep habits and time clocks. Melatonin also contains vitamin E.

PYCNOGENOL: Produced from grape seed extract and maritime pine bark, it has been said to be 50 times as potent as vitamin E. It is an antioxidant which fights off free radicals generated by foreign toxic chemicals in the blood. Some say it also reduces inflammation in joints and improves the nervous system. It also strengthens collagen, boosts the immune system, enhances metabolism, promotes healing and improves circulation.

RICE BRAN EXTRACT: Three elements in the polyphenols of rice bran have a form of vitamin E that is 6,000 times as strong as the usual form of vitamin E. If the experts are right, this supplement would do wonders for all the things vitamin E does. It helps lung metabolism, increases capillary wall strength, aids muscle and nerve maintenance, and works hard as a detoxifier and immune system booster.

COENZYME Q-10: This one is a powerful antioxidant that is compared with vitamins A, C, and E. It is a benefit for fibromyalgia patients. It aids in the oxygenation of cells and tissues. It is estimated to be 20 times as strong as vitamin E. It boosts biochemical ability and activates cell energy as it also improves circulation. One expert says that Coenzyme Q-10 doubled the immune system's ability to clear invading organisms from the blood.

DHEA: An adrenal hormone. It is valuable as the mother hormone of the body and is good at helping to prevent osteoporosis, diabetes, high cholesterol and other immune disorders including fibromyalgia. It is also believed to be able to slow and even reverse the aging process.

L-CARNITINE: This is an amino acid that helps to breakdown fats and sugars for energy. It is effective with fibromyalgia patients because it can boost energy levels.

BEE POLLEN: Nature's most complete food. It has most of the minerals and vitamins we need. It helps fibromyalgia patients since it will increase appetite, normalize intestinal activity, strengthen capillary walls, and is the most powerful immune booster we have.

GLUCOSAMINE: Holds the key to the number of water holding molecules that form in cartilage. It has also been used to reduce sensitivity and pain in soft issue areas of fibromyalgia patients.

RECENT STUDY ON BENEFITS OF MAGNESIUM AND MALIC ACID

A recent study published in the *Journal of Nutritional Medicine* revealed that taking a combination of magnesium and malic acid showed great promise as a remedy for fibromyalgia.

Fifteen participants took 1200 to 2400 mg of malic acid with 100 to 600 mg of magnesium for a period of 4 to 8 weeks. All patients reported dramatic pain relief within 2 days.

Malic acid is a natural substance found in apples and other fruit. Because of its high concentration in apples, malic acid is often called "apple acid."

Your local health food stores will carry several products containing appropriate combinations of these two nutrients. Many of these products will have "fibro" in the name. Ask your health food store representative for information on the various brand names.

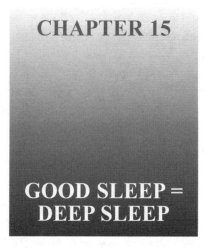

CHAPTER 15

GOOD SLEEP = DEEP SLEEP

Most of you who are suffering with fibromyalgia have some kind of sleep problem. You might have trouble getting to sleep. You may wake up at night for no reason and can't get back to sleep. You may wake yourself up snoring. You may twist and turn for hours, only to get to sleep just before your alarm goes off.

This is what doctors call non-restorative sleep. In short, it doesn't do what sleep is supposed to do: restore your body from its day's labor and rejuvenate you and mend the little nicks and tears in your system from the day before. This means your bad sleep doesn't lessen any of your muscle pain nor do anything to ease your constant feeling of fatigue.

JUST WHAT IS SLEEP?

Sleep is self-initiated unconsciousness. It all happens in the brain—the part doctors call the hypothalamus. This part of your head controls your body clock (waking and sleeping cycles) as well as thirst, sexual arousal and your appetite. Those waking and sleeping cycles are the ones we're interested in right now. Specific nerve cells in your hypothalamus dictate your waking/sleeping cycles.

You've heard that your brain is an electrical organ, dealing with things like neurotransmitters, neutron nerve cells, and our old friend serotonin. How does it all work?

The neurotransmitters carry electrical impulses from the brain along tracks in the nervous system. The nerve cells manufacture these neurotransmitters from our daily nutrition. Serotonin is one of the big guns in controlling your sleep.

Your nerve cells are not bunched together—they are separated from each other by spaces called synapses. Here is the gist of it all: Your brain says lift your arm. It sends messages to your arm through your nerve cells, one to the next, across the synapses, using those neurotransmitters we talked about. Each nerve cell takes in a chemical or electrical signal and kicks out a neurotransmitter into the synaptic space next to it. It reaches the next cell where it is boosted along to the next until it comes to the arm muscle, which is ordered to contract—you lift your arm. All this takes place in the blink of a widget's eyeball. Electricity travels fast.

So what does this have to do with your poor sleep? Lots. Those of you who have nonrestorative sleep problems add up to a little over 80 percent of FMS patients. Any input to the brain during this sleep from outside sources will further damage your good and deep sleep. If noises, movement or even lights bother you, why not try earplugs and eye masks to help shade out those problems?

Those electrical charges we talked about to lift your arm also function as you get ready to go to sleep. Same action, different paths. So let's see what kind of sleep the experts in that field tell us there are.

TWO TYPES OF SLEEP

You've probably heard of REM. That stands for Rapid Eye Movement. This stage of your sleep involves the rapid movement of your eyes, as if you were watching a movie or a tennis match. REM sleep is usually what happens after you have been sleeping for an hour to an hour and a half. Specialists can tell you are having REM by the use of electrodes attached to your head to measure brain activity and to your eyelids to measure your eye movement.

REM will result in a small rise in your temperature, and increased blood flow to the brain. This is entirely normal. Sleep experts say that they can track this activity with the use of the EEG (ElectroEncephaloGram). They think that REM sleep is connected to the storing of information and data in your long-term memory. This is also when most of your dreaming happens, although you may have REM later during the night and even wake up with a dream fresh in your conscious mind. The sleep experts say that the first REM session may last for from five to 20 minutes.

There are four different levels of normal sleep, non-REM. The first one happens when you are falling asleep. It can be a drowsy period and what the sleep folks call twilight sleep. The EEG machine will show rapid alpha waves in your brain but there is no REM. This type sleep passes quickly, usually after five or six minutes.

The next stage of your sleep is a little deeper than the first, and your brain wave activity and your breathing both start to slow down. Some say that the third stage of sleep is really an extension of the second type. Now your slow delta waves increase as your brain activity slows and cools and the brain's blood flow diminishes.

The last stage of non-REM sleep is called by some deep sleep. Here the delta waves slow down again and the period can last from thirty-five to forty minutes. This deep sleep is when your body has a chance to prop up its defenses, rebuild any damage that happened during the day in normal wear and tear, and to give your brain a rest as well. Restorative sleep is the most important kind for FMS patients. It gives your body time to fight those muscle pains, find the cause and repair a small piece of the problem. It gives your whole body a total rest period, so you can wake up in the morning refreshed and not feeling like you were dragged through a chicken coop screaming and wailing all night.

Yes, this cycle of REM and then non-REM stages is repeated several times during the night. That's why you can wake up with one dream at 2 A.M., get back to sleep and have another dream before morning. Or perhaps several dreams. So far sleep psychologists have found no connection between dreams and good or bad sleep.

WHY DO FMS PATIENTS HAVE SLEEP PROBLEMS?

Some doctors are now saying that they believe that the sleep problems are a result of a neurochemical imbalance. This same imbalance is also a big factor in muscle pain. If you are one of those FMS patients who have trouble getting to seep—then awaken often during the night and have trouble getting back to sleep—it's probably because of this neurochemical problem. Often this sleep pattern leaves the person as tired when they get up as when they went to bed. The proof seems to be that on those rare nights when they sleep through and get a good deal of deep sleep, they awaken more refreshed and even with less muscle pain.

We talked about delta waves above. Those are the good ones. Some FMS patients who have trouble sleeping have alpha waves that invade their sleep pattern where they are not supposed to be—in stages one and three and four of non-REM sleep. This causes more problems with bad sleep or not enough good sleep.

Serotonin seems to be the key here to much of the problem. Serotonin is one of those neurotransmitters that helps regulate your sleep patterns. In almost all of FMS patients, there is not enough serotonin in the blood stream to regulate the sleep patterns correctly.

THE GROWTH HORMONE STORY

Doctors now believe that the lack of delta, or deep, sleep can lead to a deficiency of the growth hormone in your body. This lack of growth hormone is thought to be at the root of many of the symptoms of fibromyalgia. Your pituitary gland produces growth hormone 24 hours a day—however, it is during deep sleep when 80 percent of this hormone is secreted into the body.

As you are painfully aware, most people with FMS simply can't get enough deep sleep. Researchers tell us that as soon as most FMS patients achieve deep sleep, they are immediately invaded by alpha waves—this destroys the deep sleep and cuts the production of growth hormone.

The result is that FMS patients are light sleepers and awaken easily, and then often have trouble getting back to sleep. This starts an unending cycle of lack of sleep and low growth hormone secretion, which leads to several fibromyalgia problems, which gets back to our lack of sleep and low growth hormone production.

Yes, you can be tested for the amount of growth hormone in your system by checking the level of somatomedin-C in your blood after the hormone breaks down. The usual result is that FMS patients have less of the somatomedin-C factor in their blood than normal. This indicates that there was less growth hormone secreted into your body.

Growth hormone is essential to adults. During regular work and walking and living, your body develops microscopic tears and fissures in your muscles in all parts of your system. Growth hormone is one of the elements in your body that helps repair these small rips. Without the right amount of this hormone, FMS patients experience muscle tightness and then pain. Another job growth hormone has is the ability to carry away from the muscles the normal amount of lactic acid that is built up there during exercises. Getting these substances away from the muscles means the body can expel them so they don't fatigue the muscles.

Not getting enough deep sleep can also damage your immune system. Your deep sleep helps in the production in your body of chemical substances called antibodies that can destroy many of the common infections. Without deep sleep, FMS patients may be more susceptible to common colds and virus illnesses.

OTHER SLEEP PROBLEMS

Insomnia is a problem for many FMS sufferers. They either

can't get to sleep when going to bed, or they sleep a little and then wake up and can't get back to sleep. When this happens the patient often gets up and paces the floor or reads or watches some TV hoping to get sleepy. After two or three hours they may get back to sleep only to awaken a few hours later grouchy and still as tired as when they went to bed.

Another sleep problem is sleep apnea. This situation is common in one quarter of FMS patients. Here the person simply stops breathing for ten to sixty seconds at various times during the night. This can have a physical cause that is not limited to FMS patients. The cause can be fatty tissue at the base of the tongue or even the tongue itself that partially blocks the air path.

This problem can often be solved by simply changing the position when you go to sleep which reduces the pressure in that area. There are some assisted breathing aids or, as the last resort, surgery to correct the cause. Sleep apnea can put a sudden strain on the heart, lungs and diaphragm when breathing resumes. This alone is enough to destroy any chance for deep sleep, and aggravates the resulting problems.

Snoring is another problem for many, and especially harmful for FMS patients. Your own loud snoring can wake you up and destroy any deep sleep you may have attained. Snoring by a spouse can also destroy your good sleep.

Snoring is sometimes caused by excess throat tissue partially blocking the air passage. Sometimes snoring increases with the use of some medications. Check your own. There are specially designed pillows to hold your head in a position to reduce snoring. As a last resort, you might want to use soft, foam earplugs: the kind you squeeze thin and insert in your ear and they expand back to their regular size. This cuts off about one third of the noise and often lets you sleep right through your own and your spouse's snoring. As a final solution, you can have excess tissue surgically removed from the throat.

Here are some more ideas to help with snoring:

1. Find the type of earplugs that men who operate noisy machinery use. Some of these are excellent. There are

several sizes and they have adjustable rings and baffles. They will cut out up to 80 percent of outside noise.

2. Try a "white sound" machine in your bedroom. These emit a soothing signal that tends to block out other sounds. Some have different sounds such as ocean surf, rain or soft music. They can work wonders. Electronic stores often stock them.

3. Talk about it with your spouse. Are you snoring or is your spouse? Figure out what to do to solve the problem. Don't blame anyone: fix it.

4. Drinking alcohol before bedtime can increase the chances and level of snoring.

5. Nudging or touching a partner who snores will often stop it. But this may have to be done every two or three minutes. The idea is to change the air intake pattern. Sometimes gently moving a quilt over the snorer's open mouth or nose will solve the problem—until that person turns and the quilt comes off.

6. Anti snoring aids such as the Breathe-Rite strips are now on the market. They are U-shaped bandages that are supposed to keep the nasal passages open. They can work.

7. If sinus problems or allergies are causing the snoring, use an antihistamine or decongestant before bedtime. This might do the trick.

8. Overly dry weather, or low humidity in the bedroom, can also lead to snoring by almost anyone. Check the humidity in your bedroom and, if it's too low, think about a humidifier to use in the bedroom.

Some fifteen percent of patients with FMS also have a condition that produces an unconscious jerking of the arms and legs. For light sleepers, this is enough to rouse them from sleep with the problem of trying to get back to sleep. It also can mean a problem maintaining a deep sleep. For this one there is a medication called clonazepam. It is an anticonvulsant, and usually stops the jerking.

Do you grind your teeth at night? About 15 percent of

fibromyalgia patients do. This usually results in morning neck or jaw pain, and your dentist will tell you it also grinds down your teeth. There are devices your dentist can show you that can slow or prevent teeth grinding. See him. Teeth grinding is often enough to wake up a light sleeper with FMS.

SOME IDEAS TO HELP YOU GET TO SLEEP AND STAY ASLEEP

ESTABLISH A ROUTINE BEFORE YOU GO TO BED. It might be listening to the late news, having a cup of caffeine-free tea, doing some light weight training such as with a stretch tube, maybe reading a chapter of a book in your favorite chair. Then to bed. Your mind and body will begin to settle into the routine and you'll find yourself winding down, ready for sleep.

WORK ON YOUR EXERCISE PROGRAM DURING THE DAY. Regular exercise—especially aerobics such as walking, bike riding, and swimming—helps tire your body so it wants to get that healing rest.

It helps. Compare your sleep habits after exercise days and when you don't have your regular workout.

FUNCTION ON A REGULAR SCHEDULE FOR GETTING TO BED AND GETTING UP. If it's ten P.M. into bed and up at six every morning, maintain those hours. The longer you stick to a schedule, the better your sleep patterns will be and the easier it is to fall asleep.

SOUNDPROOF YOUR BEDROOM. This is a great idea if you are in a noisy area such as near a freeway or an airport. Loud noises during the night affect your sleep quality, even if they don't awaken you.

Keep track of your sleep rhythms. For a month, write on your bedroom calendar when you got to sleep and when you awoke. You might also want to jot down other elements, such as any caffeine intake, your exercise, or any late night stimuli (except sex).

LET IN SOME FRESH AIR. Open the window on a cold night? Our grandparents always did. Said it helped them sleep. An overly warm room may make getting to sleep harder, but there is no proof that a cold room helps you get to sleep easier.

GET RID OF THE STIMULANTS. If you have a serious problem getting to sleep, eliminate all caffeine, alcohol, tobacco and nasal decongestants. They will keep you awake. Even chocolate has caffeine in it. Caffeine drinks can stimulate your system for up to 20 hours. Caffeine can seriously deplete your level of neurotransmitters.

TOO HUNGRY TO GET TO SLEEP? Happens to some people. They respond with a late evening snack of fruit or carbohydrate. It can help. Warm milk increases serotonin levels.

If you have trouble getting to sleep, try eating a lighter dinner and larger lunches to balance out your diet. A heavy meal at eight or nine o'clock will rev up your digestive system and can upset your sleep timing. Even a heavy meal at six can lead to sleep problems.

SHIFT GEARS. If you wake up in the middle of the night and can't get back to sleep, don't thrash around in the sheets. Get up and do something else for a while. Read a book, watch a late night TV movie, or check the 24-hour news channel. Try a light snack or four ounces of cold water. Then give the rack another try.

RELAX FIRST. Try to do a few relaxation routines before bedtime or when you wake up in the night. Consciously relax your muscles, starting at your head and neck and working down to your toes. Let the tensions drain out of you. To help learn how, there are audiotapes to train you.

RESERVE YOUR BED FOR ITS INTENDED PURPOSES. Do not read in bed. Do not watch TV while in bed. Do not eat your evening meal in bed. Your bed should be used only for sleeping, and for sex.

WARM UP. If nothing else seems to help, start taking a short, hot shower or tub bath just before bed. This will raise your body temperature and help you get to sleep.

SAVE SLEEP FOR NIGHTTIME. Do not take naps during the day unless your fatigue is debilitating. Save sleeping for nighttime and sleep will come quicker.

STAY IN THE DARK. If there is too much light in your room, or early morning light bothers you, try eyeshades or a sleep mask.

SILENCE IS GOLDEN. If noise is a problem, get yourself some earplugs and use them. Amazing what a difference they make.

Put an end to potty stops. Avoid needing to get up to urinate by cutting off any fluid intake after six P.M. Take medications that cause frequent urination in the morning, not at night.

DRESS APPROPRIATELY. Be sure your bed wear is comfortable and not binding. Use flannel sheets in the winter and sleep on a good foam rubber pad. If you use an electric blanket, try turning it on a half hour before bedtime, then turn it off when you get in bed.

USE PAIN MEDICATION WHEN NECESSARY. If nighttime pain awakens you, talk with your doctor about getting a new medication to moderate or eliminate it.

TEST A WATERBED. Would a waterbed be more comfortable and help you sleep? Don't scoff until you try one. Test a waterbed in a hotel or motel. If you get one, no matter the climate, be sure to get one with a heater. Cold in any form is bad for fibromyalgia patients.

PILLOW TROUBLE? Try a cervical pillow to support your head and neck in better alignment and reduce neck pain. If you sleep on your side, remember to have a high enough pillow to support your head on a good alignment. Don't let it drop down to your pillow.

YOUR MATTRESS? Most FMS patients do best on a foam pad of three to five inches on top of a firm mattress. To firm up the mattress, put a sheet of half-inch plywood under the mattress and on top of the box springs.

COLD FEET? Often this can awaken a light sleeper. Go ahead and put on stockings for the night. These can be anklet types or a man's longer, heavier socks—nothing binding.

USE EXTRA PADDING. Try out an egg-crate type foam pad as used in hospitals. They are readily available.

RELIEF FOR A SORE NECK MIGHT HELP SLEEPING. A bath towel rolled up and put inside a pillowcase may do the trick.

Use it under your neck to relieve some types of neck pain.

STOP HOT FLASHES. For hot flashes during the night, talk to your doctor about an estrogen replacement medication. Hot flashes can keep you awake and make your FMS symptoms worse.

MEDICATIONS TO HELP YOU SLEEP

When all else fails, talk to your doctor about a medication to help you sleep. Over-the-counter sleeping aids usually won't help you.

Most doctors prescribe a mild antidepressant drug in small doses to help FMS patients to sleep. The result usually is more restorative sleep for the patient.

Getting the right medication in the right dosage can be a problem for you and your doctor. Too much and you'll have the side effect of being drowsy during the day. Most FMS patients are given the child's dosage, but even that is too much sometimes. Then you can use your pill cutter and take what may be a quarter of a standard dose.

Work closely with your doctor. Sometimes it takes very small doses of two different medications working together to return you to deep sleep which will help fight your other FMS symptoms.

Some of the medications that are often used for aiding FMS sufferers to get to sleep include these:

ELAVIN: an amitriptyline usually used as an antidepressant. A tricyclic agent that helps slow down the reabsorption of serotonin in the nerve terminals. Effective in aiding in deep sleep.

DOXEPIN: a tricyclic agent and antihistamine with a strong sedative effect.

NORTRIPTYLINE: another tricyclic sedating drug similar to amitriptyline.

TAGAMET AND ZANTAC: anti-ulcer medications. They also block the absorption of the stimulating neurotransmitter histamine and aid with producing deep sleep. Tagamet in lower strength is now an over-the-counter drug.

PAXIL: is a specific serotonin inhibitor that creates its own pain-relieving effect for FMS patients.

ALPDRAZOLAM: an anti-anxiety drug that can increase slow wave sleep—and that's good.

CARISOPRODOL: quiets the nervous system. Should be used in the smallest dosage. Can put patients in a meditative state.

BENADRYL: an over-the-counter medication. It's used as an antihistamine and for allergies. It makes many people drowsy and may help you sleep.

MELATONIN: a hormone secreted at nightfall by the pineal gland. Its job is to make you feel sleepy. Now available as a supplement in some health food stores. Some people who use it get depressed. Experiments are now being done to see if melatonin in large doses can be used for birth control.

CALMS FORTE: a homeopathic formula to help you sleep— available in health food stores.

THE FINAL LAST RESORT

If nothing else works for you, your final step in getting sleep relief is to be tested in a sleep laboratory. Ask your doctor where one is available, and to recommend one he's worked with. After a number of tests, the specialist and your doctor can tailor a program for you. Often these centers will want you to sleep in the lab for two nights. Some labs will set up a test in your home, bringing in their equipment. This way they can get your sleep patterns in your normal surroundings so there is no skewing of the results.

CHAPTER 16

COPING WITH FIBROMYALGIA AT HOME

Coping is a great word. Most of us know in general what it means. Look at it this way: "Cope: to face and deal with responsibilities or problems calmly and adequately." That's a great definition. Since most of you reading this are women, let's look at how many women must deal with their responsibilities.

COOKING, FOOD, CLEAN-UP

Probably one of the biggest problems that faces a woman with fibromyalgia is cooking. This true for anyone, but if you work full time, cooking becomes a double chore. With your fibromyalgia it can turn into a daily horror scene.

There are ways you can cope with cooking and food preparation and cleanup. If you had always thought of cooking dinner as the crowning achievement of the day, it's time to reevaluate the whole scene. Many women with FMS find they can't stand for long periods of time to do fancy desserts and complicated meals. Why not scale down your menu? Easy-to-fix casseroles and simple salads can serve well. Try some of the prepared dinners for one meal a week. Think what foods are nourishing and healthy and at the same time easy to fix.

If you have older children, bring them into the meal preparation process. It will be instructive to them, and at the same time keep you off your feet and out of pain as they help out in the food preparation.

Some ideas about how you can cope with the cooking syndrome and still not mess up your pain level.

1. Instead of slaving over individual servings, lay out a salad bar on your counter top. Put out various kinds of lettuce, green onion, sliced beets, cheese, carrots, sprouts, tomatoes, nuts, raisins, croutons and anything else you need for a salad and three kinds of salad dressing. Let your family or guests then make their own salad. It works.

    You can do the same thing for tacos. Put out all of the ingredients and the warm taco shells and the taco sauce and it's a simple meal. You can cut and grate the elements while sitting at the kitchen table. The refried beans and the hamburger cook and heat up quickly on the stove.

2. Concentrate on foods with multiple uses. For example, cook a big stew that can last for at least two meals. Same idea for a good- sized roast that can work for two or three meals and sandwiches in the mean time. A roasting chicken is another good multiple meal idea that can produce the first meal, then chicken salad, hot chicken sandwich or even chicken a la king the third night. Or freeze some of the chicken for quick microwave warmup later on.

3. The microwave is a godsend for easy cooking these days. For warming up leftovers it's a marvel. For fast cooking foods, it is great. The average sized potato will bake in a microwave at high in six to eight minutes. The same spud in your conventional oven will take 45 minutes. Always think fast for your cooking. The faster you can cook, the quicker you get off your feet.

4. In one way slow is good: the good old crock pot slow cooker. Get it started in the morning or early noon for the four to six-hour cook before dinner. Easy prepara-

tion, no standing/stove watching.

5. Leftovers can become meals. Save those cup or two-cup sized leftovers and put them in plastic tubs and store them in your freezer compartment. When you get enough leftovers, you might be able to use one of those microwave plastic meal trays and combine them into a good meal. Another idea is to drop them in a pot with some leftover roast or turkey and a can of stewed tomatoes and make a great soup.

6. When you do your measuring, mixing and stirring, try to do it next to the sink. Then if you spill anything, it is easier to clean up than if it were on the stove or the table.

7. Are your best hours in the morning? Do your basic set-up then. Most foods can be warmed up deliciously. Say you're doing a steak dinner. Cook your potatoes and gravy and vegetables, then put them in the refrigerator. The steak you'll do just before serving. But you've cut your evening workload by two thirds.

8. Does grating cheese hurt your hands and arms? Try freezing small sections of cheese. When you thaw it out, most kinds will crumble in your hand. Saves the work.

9. If you have older kids, set up one night a week when the kids get to cook the meal, or cook just for themselves. To facilitate this program, be sure you have on hand plenty of fast foods: sandwich fixings, chili, hot dogs and frozen burger patties, and any leftover casseroles, roasts or chicken. Make it easy for them.

In your mother's day, the woman of the house took great pride and satisfaction in providing delicious and nutritious meals for her family. That was her main job. These days many men love to cook—don't shut out your spouse. Let him be an even partner in the cooking/kitchen work.

CREATIVE KITCHEN PLANNING

Most kitchens are built to be used by people who stand up. Many times, fibromyalgia patients have trouble standing for even short periods of time. You can solve part of this problem by finding the right height stool to use at your sink and counter and stove. Look at bar and stool places and in used furniture stores. Then you can sit down at the counter—sideways, granted, but it will take the strain off your legs and back.

Another way to work on the standing up problem is to do all of the cooking preparation you can while sitting in a chair at the kitchen table. Bring what you need to the table. If you're cutting up vegetables for a soup or a stew or getting ready to make stuffing for a chicken or turkey, the kitchen table is a good alternative to the sink or counter top.

When you have to stand at your sink or counter, get an eight or ten inch high footstool and put one foot on it when you work at the sink. This will change your balance and be restful for your back and aching muscles. Alternate the foot on the stool.

Another small suggestion. Sit near the sink and try pulling out a drawer near it that you can put a cutting board across. Use this for cutting, chopping, preparation for baking, etc. Depending on your kitchen set up, this could be extremely helpful.

A wide-based stool that will get you up to the counter that comes with rollers on it will also prove helpful. Then you can roll from one spot to another the way people do in offices. Be sure the stool has a wide base for stability.

SOME KITCHEN CLEANUP IDEAS

Let your dishwasher get full before you turn it on. It doesn't save much time or effort, but it seems to be more efficient to run the dishwasher once every two days, rather than every day.

When you empty the dishwasher, put everything on the counter top. Then sit down and put away the silver in the drawer. For dishes and glasses on the shelves, take a step or two up on your step stool so you don't have to lift things so high. Helps.

If there are only two or three of you for meals, serve directly from the cooking pots to the plates, then take the plates to the table. Saves putting food into serving dishes, and saves the work of washing and putting them away.

GROCERY SHOPPING

Shopping for groceries is really an aerobic exercise. It's easy to spend from a half-hour to an hour walking up and down the aisles of a huge shopping market. There are a few ideas to help you. If shopping is the longest walk you ever take, try to handle the job by using a motorized rig with the cart in front. Many grocery supermarkets now offer these to customers.

If you can use one, don't be bashful about climbing on board and start shopping. They are convenient and useful for those who can't walk well or not at all. People in wheel chairs usually don't use them because they can be hard to get in and out of.

Your store doesn't have such a convenience? Talk with the manager, and explain your physical condition and ask him to get such a rig. Remind him there probably are a number of people in his store who would appreciate having one to use.

It is especially important for you to have a shopping list. Check your list as you start at one end of the store and work up and down the aisles to the far end. Look over your list on every aisle so you don't have to backtrack.

If you don't know where an item is, ask a clerk or stocker to go get one for you. Most supermarkets bend over backwards on this score to help customers.

As a further convenience, you may wish to label the food shelves with little name tags: stewed tomatoes, beans, peaches, chicken gravy or soups. When you make out your shopping list, you can see what space is vacant and know you need at least one can of that one.

Also keep a list on your refrigerator of what you need. When you run out of onions, mark it on the paper and have that paper ready when you make out your shopping list.

CLEANING YOUR HOME

Just how clean does clean have to be? Let's say you live with your husband and no children are home. How clean should your house be? Before FMS you may have had a strict schedule of mopping, dusting, doing the curtains and vacuuming. Let's be practical. You can't do all those things now every week. No one with white gloves is going to be inspecting your place.

Cut down your list to the essentials. What must be done? How often? Where can you cut the workload? The bathroom and the kitchen are the most important. Germs can kill you. Now look at your cleaning schedule again. Make a list for once a week, once every two weeks, and then "whenever you get to it."

Don't get paranoid about cleaning. Do what you are physically able to do and try not to worry about the rest. If your husband is the helpful type, have a talk and explain your situation. He probably will help. If not, then do what you can, when you can. Remember it isn't a contest. Here are some ideas that may help:

1. A cluttered room always looks messy and dirty. Start by cleaning up the clutter. Put it out of sight or throw it away. Keep in the living room what you need to be there and what looks good.

2. Work on one room at a time. For example, don't dust the whole house. Dust, vacuum, arrange, and polish one room at a time and it will be looking good. Then quit and don't worry about the rest of the house.

3. Watch your strength level. If you start getting tired when half way through a job, don't worry—take a break. Maybe you'll come back to that dusting job the next day. Remember, nobody with white gloves will inspect your house.

4. Ever thought of singing while you work? Or even whistling, as the song goes. Nobody is listening. Sing those old favorites of the forties, fifties, sixties, and seventies. Singing will make the time go faster and you'll feel better at the same time.

5. For dusting those ceiling corners and high walls, use a

long-handled duster. Keeps you from reaching so far. Try dusting the TV screen first with your synthetic duster. It will pick up an electrical static charge from the tube, and dust in many other places will now stick to the material until you give it a good shaking outside.

6. Never overdo. If you feel that you're getting tired, don't push for five more minutes to finish a job. Nobody is watching. Always quit working on that cleaning job when you can still do a little more. That will be good for you. There's always tomorrow, Scarlett.

LAUNDRY: ALWAYS A PROBLEM

For most women with serious FMS, the weekly wash is usually a big hurdle to get over. Just gathering the clothes and bedding to be washed and dried can be a forbidding task. Do you use a laundry basket? Chances are it might be as heavy as half of the clothes in it. Instead of the basket, try stuffing everything in a pillowcase or on a sheet and tie the four corners. It's a lighter bundle to carry.

Front loading washers are easier to use than the top kind. The next time you get a new washer, consider one like that. Are you tired out by the time you get the laundry gathered and to the washer? Always have a chair near your washer and dryer so you can sit down and take a rest.

No one has you on a stopwatch to see how fast you work. Take it easy. Rest a while, then put the laundry in to wash.

Getting the clothes out of a top load washer is a nearly impossible chore for FMS patients who have serious arm and shoulder pain. Do it slowly one or two pieces at a time. Simply drop them on the door of a front loading dryer. When the stack is high enough, bend down and push the items into the dryer.

Again, there is no rush. Take it easy. Rest again if you need to in that handy chair.

Lightweight, plastic laundry baskets are best. Mostly because they are so light and can hold lots of wash. When your clothes come out of the dryer, just drag them over the door and let them drop into the laundry basket just below and in front of it.

Everyone does the folding and putting away differently. Try this: take the basketful into your living room, set it near your favorite soft chair and sit down and turn on the TV. Now you can fold the clothes at leisure while you watch a soap, or an African lion documentary, or even an old movie. Do not stand up in your bedroom as you fold and sort clothes and bedding.

When you're rested, or when the show is over, you can stack the folded clothes back in the laundry basket and take them to the bedroom and put the items away.

CHAPTER 17

OVERCOMING FIBROMYALGIA AT WORK

M ost people with fibromyalgia work, just like everyone else. Most have to work to make a living. In a recent survey it was learned that only about 15 percent of FMS patients have given up trying to hold a job and do not work.

That figure should be lower. More and more FMS patients are learning how to control their symptoms, how to work through them, and how to get their daily tasks at their job done despite their pain and their individual problems.

As of 1990 there has been a law of the land called the ADA, the Americans with Disabilities Act. This law directs employers to work with a "qualified individual with a disability" and to make "reasonable accommodations," so that person can continue working.

It has been a gift from heaven for some. For others the law has been ignored by their employers and not enforced. At its best it is a good law that helps those partly disabled to stay on the job with small "accommodations" by the employer.

Generally the law refers to any individual who has a physical or mental impairment that substantially limits one or more of the person's major activities. What does that mean? If you can't lift fifteen pounds repeatedly or can't sit at a desk for a half-hour doing work, you qualify as having a physical impairment. The list of impairments runs on for pages. For the most part it includes those problems we have with FMS.

Now, what "accommodations" does your employer need to make so you can keep on working? As you can imagine, the accommodations are many and varied. Some of them might include adjusting facilities to make them more accessible to people, redefining the person's job, making changes in responsibilities, giving work the person can do, changing equipment, offering part-time work, changing work hours—almost anything that can allow the person to keep on working so he or she can still be a productive worker for the company.

If you work for someone with fewer than 15 employees, the firm does not have to follow the ADA laws. They are exempt. Some companies with more than 15 workers can be exempt for specific reasons.

Here are some fibromyalgia problems and the general type of accommodations that might be made to help. You might want to suggest some of these to your boss to help her accommodate your physical or mental situation.

FATIGUE

- Let you have more rest periods, or longer ones.
- Schedule you for more frequent rest breaks.
- Allow you to pace yourself to get your day's work done.
- Set up a place where you can lie down for a short nap or rest break.
- Get outside help to check on your workstation's ergonomics.
- Devise some type of job-sharing situation.
- Work out scheduling so you can do your work at home one day a week.
- Cut down on the amount or weight of lifting for the job.

FOR THOSE WITH MUSCLE PAIN OR STIFFNESS

- Set up a workstation where the employee can either sit or stand or alternate between the two.
- Allot special close by parking, and easy ramps to eliminate going up steps to the work place.

- Cut down on repetitive tasks, or space them out with other duties.
- Make available a suitable ergonomic workstation or chair that fits the worker's needs.
- Allow for short breaks for the worker to move around the work area to reduce same-place stiffness.

TOO HOT, TOO COLD

- Double check to see that ventilation is good and consider an air purifier.
- In extreme heat or cold, let the person work at home.
- Permit multi-layered clothing in cold situations.
- Provide a space heater or fan for this individual.
- Move the person out of direct air conditioning or heating airflow.
- If the employee has an office, allow individual heat/cool controls.

CONCENTRATION PROBLEMS

- Avoid SAD by providing additional lighting in winter months.
- Reduce loud noises from industrial areas with white sound machines, soundproofing, or sound baffles.
- Allow this employee to work at home some days a week.
- Offer more than required rest breaks.
- Confirm with worker the job requirements, and any deadlines.
- Divide large jobs into smaller parts and re-distribute to others.
- Provide calendars and memos when jobs are due.
- Give the worker uninterrupted work time and space.

STRESS OR DEPRESSION

- Initiate stress management training for all employees.
- Provide other workers who can support and mentor.
- Allow work-time appointments with medics or counselors.

BOWEL AND BLADDER CONTROL

- Locate the worker close to the bathroom.
- Don't dock the worker for time in the rest room.
- Provide leave time as needed for medical appointments and to recover from irritable bowel syndrome situations.

HEADACHES

- If a computer is used, provide a glare guard on the screen.
- Provide correct ventilation and, if needed, an air purifier.
- Filter or dim fluorescent lights if they are a problem.
- Use proper task lighting for the situation.
- Allow flexible work time scheduling if a busy office is a cause.

OTHER WORK-RELATED PROBLEMS

There are a lot of problems that come up at work for patients with FMS. We'll cover some of them here and remind you to look critically at any new strain, stress or pain you feel in your body during or just after work. It probably isn't just in your head.

CUMULATIVE TRAUMA DISORDER

This is a medical term that covers a lot of problems such as tennis elbow, carpal tunnel syndrome, tendonitis in hand or wrist, thoracic outlet syndrome, and cubital tunnel syndrome.

Office workers are often subject to these ailments, but they can also happen to musicians, stitchers and sewers, supermarket checkers, assembly line workers, even long distance drivers. Anyone who has to do much the same motion hundreds of times a day can develop some of these disorders. Patients with fibromyalgia may be especially susceptible to these ailments. If you are in one of these situations, check yourself frequently. If you develop symptoms for any of them, run—don't walk—to your doctor for a checkup.

These repetitive motion jobs mean there can be damage to the tendons, nerves, joints and muscles from the constant friction. A sedentary position, and small hand and arm movements, can also mean a lack of blood flow into the affected areas. New blood into a part of the body that is hurting is the first way the body tries to repair the damage. You can increase this blood flow by stretching and correcting your posture during your work.

- Some warning signs for repetitive strain injury:
- Numbness and tingling in your hands, arms, or fingers.
- Pain in your wrists or at the base of your thumb.
- Your grip is not as strong as it used to be.
- A new pain in your shoulders, back, or neck.
- A new clumsiness, or lack of control of arms and legs.
- A growing heaviness in your forearms and with your hands.
- Doing tasks with your left hand you usually do with your right.
- A strange, heightened awareness of one or both hands.
- Giving up a hobby or game because it hurts your hands.

These symptoms will almost surely be gradual and slip up on you without your knowing it. If you become aware of any pain or sensitivity in any of these areas, and you do repetitive work, don't wait. Contact a doctor about it at once. Your General Practitioner is the place to start. He may refer you to a specialist, but get his best advice on who might be best. Actually there isn't just one specialist who does best in this area. A neurologist would be more concerned with the nerve function in the area, not the soft tissue itself. The rheumatologist is more worried about joints and bones than the overall picture. Maybe your GP is the best bet after all.

Remember that RIS (Repetitive Injury Syndrome) is not FMS. They have no connection other than that they both can hurt terribly. Your FMS may make you more aware of a hurting body, and when a new one pops up, you should recognize it sooner and get help faster.

COMPUTERS AND FMS

If you have FMS and work on a computer on your job, there are bunches of things you should consider. Most of these you can take care of yourself without any hassle with your boss. The more relaxed and comfortable you can be in front of your screen, the more productive and helpful you'll be to your firm.

Lists of the correct way to work on a computer have been around for ten years or more. Most people don't even read them anymore, and most people make a lot of mistakes that they don't have to, which can lead to physical problems whether you have FMS or not. Look at these:

AT YOUR KEYBOARD

Sit normally in your chair in front of your keyboard. Can you look slightly above center of your screen without tilting your head or glancing upward with your eyes? If so your screen is the right height.

Is there room around your screen and keyboard for those items you need: dictionary, tissue, pen, paper for notes, etc.?

Will your legs go under your keyboard so they are parallel to the floor? Don't let them touch the keyboard platform.

Your arms should be level with the floor when you touch the keyboard. Better to be a bit high rather than too low. This helps relax your arms and shoulders.

Can you press the keys easily, without extra hand movement, to be sure the connection has been made and the letter printed on the screen?

Can you reach all the shift and function keys without strain? Do you constantly hit a second key when reaching for another, so you get a double print on the screen? Try the keyboard that's angled in a small V toward the screen. The center is also slightly raised for a more natural position.

YOUR CHAIR AND SITTING POSITION

Can you sit with your torso straight and with support on the lower back? If not, adjust to this position by moving your chair forward. You may need a rolled up towel in the small of your back for better support.

Do your feet rest flat on the floor? They should.

Your thighs should be parallel with the floor. If not, you may need to lower your chair an inch or two.

Now, do your knees bend at a right angle? They should.

If your arms are not parallel to the floor when you are working the keyboard, lower your chair until they are.

Your wrists should be parallel with the floor as well, not bent up or down.

Always rest the heel of your palm on any built-in wrist rest or special one put directly behind the keyboard. Many keyboards now come with a built-in wrist rest.

LIGHTING YOUR COMPUTER

If you work from material on a copy stand, be sure that it is at the same level as your screen. This means less eye movement to go from copy to screen. You may need to set your copyholder on a stack of books to get it up. Don't let it sit on your desktop. Also keep the copy at the same distance from your eyes as your screen.

Sit so your eyes are 18-20 inches from the screen. You may need a special pair of glasses with this focal length for best vision of the screen and your copy.

No matter what font or type size you use, set the screen zoom at "page width". This will blow up your type until it fits on the screen width, anywhere from 114 to 120 percent normal size. It makes it much easier to read on the screen. Yes, it will be the correct size for the type size you choose on your guideline when it's printed out.

Always face your screen away from your office or home windows. That way you'll get no reflection from the window. You may wish to close the blinds just in back of your screen to cut down the glare in your eyes.

Use small lamps or high intensity lamps to light your copy, your work on the desk and your keyboard, instead of glaring overhead lights. Easier on your eyes, better to see the work.

If your monitor flickers, or is blurry, order a new one. Most monitors will outlast three or four computers, but they do decay.

For easier reading, get a nineteen-inch or larger computer screen and put it on "full screen" setting.

MORE IDEAS FOR FMS PATIENTS TO USE AT THEIR COMPUTER

Place your computer near the edge of your keyboard on your dominant hand side.

Place it so you don't have to reach for the mouse.

If you don't have a commercial keyboard wrist support, fold up a hand towel lengthways twice and lay it there. Works fine.

Support your forearm when you move the mouse. Move it with your hand, not your whole arm.

There are keyboard strokes to replace many mouse movements. Two strokes for print out, file, and spell check, dozens of them. It's always easier to make two keystrokes than to take your hand off the keyboard, find the mouse and move the cursor to the right spot and click it.

If you use your mouse a lot, check out the new ones at a computer store. They are ergonomic now, work easier, faster. Also look at the touch pads and trackballs.

Long fingernails cause a lot of typos. If you work for a living on your computer, cut the fingernails down even with the end of your fingers. Your typing speed and accuracy will jump by 20%.

GET IN A WORKOUT AT WORK

We did a whole chapter on exercising and working out. This is a bit different. Why not do some of your exercising at work? Smart people do it every day. No, don't get into your shorts, T-shirt and sneakers for these. Most of them can be done right at your desk between sips of coffee or after you finish a tough job on your computer or workstation.

Try these:

1. Look straight ahead, then shrug your shoulders up as high as you can and hold for a count of three. Then drop them down. Do this ten times.

2. Tilt your head, right ear downward toward your right shoulder as far as it will go. Stretch your neck. Hold it for a four count, then return your head upright. Now do

the same thing on your left side. Repeat both sides five to ten times.

3. Seated, let your chin lower to your chest until it touches. Hold there for three counts, then lift your chin upward as far as it will go and hold for three counts. Do this five to ten times.

4. Hands in front, elbows bent at your sides. Press both elbows behind you as far as you can and hold for a three count. Relax and bring hands back to front. Repeat five times.

5. While standing, place your hands with thumbs forward on your waist just above your hips. Lean backward as far as you can holding your hands firm. Hold five seconds, return to front. Do this ten times.

6. Seated, turn your head as far to the right as you can, looking over your shoulder. Hold three counts, then bring back front. Now do the same thing over your left shoulder. Repeat these two stretches five times.

7. Place your hands on the arms of your chair and, without using your legs, push your body upward until your arms are as straight as possible. A vertical pushup. Do this ten times.

8. Place your feet about three feet from a wall and lean in with both hands on the wall until you can touch your forehead on the wall. Now do wall pushups for as many as you can. Ten is good, fifty is great.

No, don't do all of these every day or every time you have your little mini workout. You may want to do some in the morning, others in the afternoon. Space them out. Use them to break up your work routine, especially if it's repetitive, and whenever you can squeeze them in.

CHAPTER 18

TRAVELING WITH FIBROMYALGIA

Yes, Virginia, there is travel after you are diagnosed as having fibromyalgia. After knowing what your ailment is, you may have a rush of joy finally knowing what your troubles are and that they are not just in your head. Before then, you may have had a period of thinking that your active life was over—it isn't.

Think it through again. You can do almost all of the things you used to do. Maybe you don't want to run a marathon, but you never did that. What you can do is travel. Some inconvenience? Yes. Some places you can't get to because there are 187 steps to the top of the overlook or the statue or the top of the building? Fine, take the view lower down. There will be a little adaptation, depending on just how severe your symptoms are.

I had a friend who had a serious case of multiple sclerosis, (MS). She had advanced to the point where she used a power wheel chair that someone else drove. She couldn't stand or move her legs. Her arm movements were restricted. She fed herself with extreme difficulty. The couple had always traveled. They went right on traveling.

Her husband spent six months arranging their trips down to the last detail, including lifts on trains and buses, and finding taxis in advance that could take the heavy motorized chair.

He had the schedule and the list of events that they both could attend and enjoy. Their trips went off without a hitch. Two weeks in Europe. A tour of Australia. A week on a jungle camera safari in Africa. They kept on taking the trips right up to the last year before she passed away.

You can travel.

Here are some hints and helps and ideas to make your travel easier with your FMS.

TRAVELING BY CAR

For some, leisurely traveling by car, or motor home, is the ideal way to get around and see the country and get up close and personal with the outback of America. You see so much more when driving through on secondary roads than you can by flying over it or even going by bus or train.

In a car you control your schedule. You never miss a flight. You don't have to tussle with your luggage down those endless corridors, or stuff your take-along bag in that incredibly high rack over the seats.

If you get tired, you can pull over and take a nap, or you can turn into a motel and get an early sleep. You can even sleep to noon the next day and get out just before check out time.

Yes, there are some drawbacks. You or your partner are in control of the machine. You must be alert while driving, watch for any problem ahead, learn to drive a long way ahead of yourself, and be responsible for the safety of yourself, your car and any passengers.

When driving, you need to hold your hands in about the same place for long periods of time. If that is a painful position, you need to make some adjustments. Driving instructors say hold the wheel with both hands at the ten o'clock and two o'clock positions on the wheel. Yes, best safety advice. If you find that painful, try what a long haul trucker taught me. Sit relaxed and comfortable behind the wheel, sitting tall, then grasp the bottom of the wheel with one hand, palm down. Now, you're ready to make small movements of the wheel either way. In an emergency you can slap your other hand up to turn the wheel as needed.

The middle of the bottom of the wheel is the most relaxed position your hand and arm can be in, even perched partly on your armrest or your side. Try it.

Now the seat. Most newer cars have adjustable driver seats. If yours does, you know by now where the best position is for the comfort of your body and good driving control. Be sure you don't have to tilt your head forward to see the road. Be sure you are sitting close enough to the wheel to hold it comfortably.

Can you easily reach the brake and gas pedals? If not, move the seat forward or back until you can.

You may want a pillow for your back. A rolled-up towel held together with rubber bands is excellent for your lumbar support.

One easy trick is to grasp the seat belt with your left hand as you get in the driver's seat and pull the belt in with you. Now you don't have to fumble around trying to find it over and behind your left shoulder. A little practice here and you can sit down and fasten that belt in a breeze.

Safety experts say not to drive for more than two hours without taking a break. This might be a ten-minute walk around a rest stop along the highway, or at a restaurant that beckons you with a roadside sign. Since you're not drinking caffeine, don't get a cup of coffee unless it's decaf. A carbonated non-caffeine orange or lemon-lime might perk you up a little.

Take a tip from retired folks: Take a three-day trip from Monday to Wednesday. There are fewer people and tourists on the roads then, shops and scenic areas and events are less crowded, and you can travel in a more relaxed style without all those tourists bothering you.

If you have a motor home, plan out your trip carefully to be sure you can get hookups at an RV camp. As you have discovered, finding a good place to park your big rig is a lot harder than simply pulling into one of the millions of motels along major highways. A little pre-planning will let you relax and not have the trauma of hunting for a place to stay the night. This is good advice for those traveling by car as well. If you get there early, have an early supper before the room is ready. If you get there a little late, the room will be reserved for you. This helps take the anxiety and worry out of finding a spot to stay. Many motel chains will reserve a room for you at another of their motels of your choice. It's a free service. If you like the motel you're at, the next one in the same chain will probably be similar.

If you're a passenger in the car, it's easier to sit in a comfortable position. A soft pillow may work just right to cushion your head and neck to prevent any strain. The rolled up lumbar towel in the small of your back may also come in handy.

If you're going on a longer trip, remember to allow time to stop and rest. It helps. Then you don't have to rush and hurry. Rushing often leads to accidents.

TRAVEL PLANS

When you make plans to take a trip to somewhere that's new, remember to set up your travel plans in advance. Think about the best way to get there: plane, train, or car. What hotel will you stay at? Can you guarantee to get a handicapped room if you need one? Talk to the hotel by phone and explain your limitations. Are the cafes and eating areas down steps or do they have ramps? Are there any other special facilities that you need? Does the hotel have a gym or exercise room?

Most moderately priced hotels will do everything they can to accommodate you and your special needs. Be sure to make your reservations well in advance and get a confirmation number. Write it down in your travel kit so you can prove your reservation if you need to.

Airlines are notorious for over-booking flights. This is because some people who reserve don't show up. If the flight you booked is full, let someone else volunteer to get off and delay their flight. If you need a wheelchair at the gate, be sure to ask for one. If you will need an aisle chair for boarding, tell the person at the gate check-in. This is a small chair with wheels that will roll between the airline rows of seats. A normal wheel chair will not fit in there.

If you're a non-smoker, ask for a non-smoking room. Most hotels have them now. Some have 50/50 smoke and non-smoke rooms and floors. Since you're in a foreign environment, better take your eyeshades and earplugs to help you get your required deep sleep.

Think to take anything that will add to your comfort. Some people never travel even by plane without their favorite pillow. Just don't forget and leave it in the hotel. A small flashlight, night readout clock and your supply of medications are all important to your having a good vacation.

LUGGAGE

The least you can take to keep you happy, well clothed and comfortable is the right amount. Don't take along three times as many clothes as you can wear. If you're flying, you may want to get everything in a wheeled bag that will fit in the overhead compartment. Ask the flight attendant to put it up there if it's hard or impossible for you to do.

TRAVELING BY PLANE

First, be sure that you have reservations on the plane you want to fly. Call the airport an hour before you leave for the flight to see if it is still scheduled and on time. Check the weather at your place. Could there be a killer fog out there that closed the airport? If the news says it's closed and flights are backed up, there's no need to go out there.

Have someone drive you to the airport or take one of the commercial air shuttles. These are commercial operations that pick you up at your home and stop for others on the way. Much less expensive than calling a taxi.

Allow plenty of time all around. Be sure to get to the airport an hour to an hour and a half before your flight leaves. For international flights, make that two hours.

Check your bags at the curb if you can. This will get them moving—your ticket will be inspected and you'll be told which gate your flight leaves from. Keeps you from standing in the long line of those waiting to buy tickets.

Oh, always get your ticket in hand before your travel day. Makes it much easier. Some airlines may be going to a no-ticket operation. Watch it. Not sure if it will catch on. Evidently if you're on the computer, you're allowed to go on board.

We talked about packing and luggage. One overhead bag and one under the seat ahead of you are the ideal. If you don't like the overhead, check one bag and keep all essentials in the bag under the seat with you.

If you need assistance getting on and off a plane, just ask the clerk or check-in person. Most airlines are extremely good about helping disabled folks, elders, and mothers with babies.

Many fibromyalgia patients reserve a bulkhead seat or an aisle seat so it's easier to get in and out of the seat, and to get up and move around on a long flight. It can pay off.

Food on airlines is always criticized. If you need a special diet, let the attendant know. Usually they will have a vegetarian plate. Don't look for no-sugar, no-fat meals. If you are really phobic about airline food, simply bring along a snack of your own. That way you control it absolutely.

CHANGES IN TIME ZONES

Most people aren't adversely affected by going through three time zone changes (as from one coast to another). This is because most people can vary their sleep time by three hours and feel little effect.

With fibromyalgia patients it's more critical. If you have a definite sleep time ritual, try as best you can to maintain it. You may have to condition yourself a little. If it's a three hour change, try moving your bed time forward or back—depending which way you're traveling—by a half hour a day for three days before you leave. This gives you an hour and a half make-up time. You can probably withstand an hour and a half differential in your sleep time with little effect.

If you've tried this half-hour plan and it didn't work, go to a full hour difference for the three days before you leave. Then at your destination you should be back on track.

Some experts say no matter which way you're headed, try to take a good walk in the sun before you leave and after you arrive. Some say a three-hour sun-walk. That would be enough to put most of us in the hospital. More realistic is a half-hour stroll and then sit in the sun for an hour. The sunlight helps adjust your internal time clock. Oh, most important: don't forget to move your watch ahead or backward, depending on which way you go.

DISABLED PARKING

Some of the better laws passed in most states recently to aid fibromyalgia patients are those covering disabled parking (DP). If you need a disabled permit, apply for it. Usually states require a doctor's written statement why you should have such a placard. Any ailment that involves walking is usually enough.

Don't be bashful about getting or using a disabled card if you need one. If some days you find it tough to walk fifty feet without taking a rest, tell your doctor. For those of you who are marginally disabled (fine sometimes, hurting others) make it an ironclad rule that you use the placard only on those days that you absolutely must have it.

If you need a cane or a walker, use them when you need to along with the placard, so you can park closer to your destination.

Most states give you your choice of using a placard you hang on your rearview mirror or put on the dash, or a license plate with a disabled icon. Both have advantages. If you ride in other people's cars often, the placard can be taken from car to car. The placard is for you, not for your car. So it can be used in any car that you're riding in.

On the other hand, you never forget to display the disabled parking notification when it's on your license plate.

In most states you apply for the placard or plate at the same agency that issues your drivers license and auto registration. Most are cooperative.

Caution: Never misuse your DP placard. Don't use it when

you don't absolutely need it. Never loan it out to someone else to use.

Don't park in a disabled spot unless you display your placard. In some states the fine for parking in a DP marked parking spot without a placard showing is $350.

TRAVELER AID IDEAS

Always carry a plastic bottle of water with you when you travel. Use one you can refill. Never be caught without some water. Then you won't have to buy coffee or a carbonated drink.

On trips, wear your athletic walking shoes. They will give you the most comfort and best traction in case of wet or slippery footing.

Ride the electric passenger cart at the airport. Wait a minute to get on one. Ask an airport clerk or attendant to help you find one and to tell you how to get where you need to go.

On a plane, put one of their small pillows in the middle of your back for better lumbar support.

Don't try to walk too far or to too many tourist haunts. You'll pay for it the next day. Take your time. Come back and finish the walk the next day.

Be sure to carry all the medications you'll need. It's almost impossible to get original prescriptions filled in foreign countries.

You'll dehydrate on a long airline flight. Ask the attendant for sparkling water or non-caffeine soda. Avoid coffee and alcoholic drinks which worsen your dehydration.

Can't sleep at your destination? Try 3 to 6 mg of melatonin. It will help you get to sleep until you acclimatize to the new time.

Dress comfortably for travel. Dressing too well invites pickpockets and confidence men. Loose clothing and athletic shoes or flats are best.

If you get added muscle pain from walking or exercising on vacation, use some ibuprofen to moderate that pain.

Set aside some time each day to take it easy. Read your

favorite book, or use a relaxation tape.

Always try for non-stop flights between destinations. Changing planes is a hassle. If non-stops are not available, often one stop with no change of planes can be booked.

Thinking about a cruise? The largest cruise ships have ramps and elevators as well as handicapped staterooms. Most handicapped rooms are three times as large as regular rooms.

If you rent a car, get one with all-power accessories and with cruise control for ease of traveling.

In your travel kit, take along a brief medical history and all of the medications that you use. If you're going overseas, find out what the equivalent names of your medications are in that country. Your pharmacist probably can help you out.

Take along the names and phone numbers of your doctors. Just in case you need to contact one of them.

CHAPTER 19

LIVING WITH FIBROMYALGIA ON A PERSONAL LEVEL

Living with fibromyalgia is an intensely personal issue, physically, mentally and socially. It is not simple or easy. You didn't ask for this condition. Nothing you did or didn't do brought it upon you. There no easy way to get rid of the syndrome of pains, problems and conditions.

For the best living experience, you must walk a tightrope between taking care of your physical needs and pains, and satisfying your emotional needs.

If you have daily pain, fatigue and bouts with depression, it's terribly difficult to keep a good attitude and to do the things you need to do to help maintain your best possible health—and remain sane and well balanced at the same time.

AFTER YOUR DIAGNOSIS

For some, the firm diagnosis that you have fibromyalgia comes as a welcome relief. You now understand that you don't have some mysterious sudden death type disease, and that your pains and problems aren't all in your head.

You have something solid and tangible that you can get a bite out of, know what is happening in your body, and understand what it takes to make you better. If you had problems sleeping and had the connected muscle pains and fatigue, you now can understand the genesis of these problems.

At the same time you know for sure now that there is going to be a big change in your life style. If your FMS brings with it serious pains and other problems, it might mean the end of some of the activities that you have long loved. Maybe tennis is impossible now, bowling might be out, the annual dance review at your club—all sorts of physical activities that you love to do may have to be put on hold or cancelled out for good.

This alone is enough to give some people depression. Their lives are changing and they now know why, but still they can't go back to doing all the things they used to love to do.

The experts tell us that focusing too much on the problems and pains and symptoms we have often leads us into negative thinking, and that almost surely will lead to some level of depression. Instead we need to concentrate on the solutions and treatments and small victories that we have over FMS. One victory can lead to another and—with lots of hard work and the proper medications and support—we can lift out of the sorry feeling and get back on a positive note. One patient said every morning she woke up and gritted through the pain and fatigue and made a list of all the good and fun and interesting things that she could still do. It perked up her whole day.

The whole-person involvement for a FMS patient depends on how severe the symptoms are. Some have little pain and some sleep problems and that's it. They solve the sleep problem with the right medication. The deep sleep then lightens the muscle pain and they can go back to doing almost everything they could before.

For those with more severe pains, fatigue, tough sleep problems and other difficulties, there will be greater personal mental and emotional trauma.

With a severe case of fibromyalgia, there are the four stages of any serious loss: first denial, then anger, followed by depression and at last acceptance of life the way it is. These are the same stages that a survivor goes through after the death of a loved one.

A person with a hard case of FMS does suffer considerable loss. Look at it this way: you suffer the loss of energy to participate in your usual activities. You lose certain roles in your family life. You lose recreational games and sports. You lose your independence. You lose financial security due to medical expenses.

You may lose the ability to enjoy sex. You lose your ability to contribute to worthwhile causes. You may lose your job and suffer a loss of income.

When some or all of these hit a person with FMS, there is bound to be a strong reaction by the patient. You will go into denial.

DENIAL

This is almost automatic with people when anything devastating happens. It has been called a protection device for the mind, until the person can become aware of the whole situation. Denial might turn up in your refusal to believe that you can't do everything you used to—until you try, and hurt yourself or become fatigued and furious. Denial must be worked through gradually until the person can realistically understand the situation at hand.

ANGER

Once over the denial stage, anger surfaces. You're mad at everyone and everything. You hate the doctor who diagnosed you. You're angry with the nurse who gives you advice and prescriptions. You're upset at the people who don't understand what FMS is and how it affects you. The anger stage may last only a short time, as the patient soon realizes that the anger is doing no good, and surely can't help to fight the problems that you have.

Don't seal up the anger inside you. Find some non-violent way of getting it out. Talk things through with your spouse, or doctor. Boil over and get it over with and then move on to the next stage.

DEPRESSION

Too often the next stage of a serious loss due to FMS can be depression. It's a natural response to this sudden cutback in the activities that you've been doing for years and love to do. Maybe you can't sing in the choir anymore because you can't stand up that long to practice, and you can't process into the church and up the steps into the choir loft. That's depressing.

Depression in its worst stages can turn off a person so they do nothing, hear nothing, or don't want to get out of bed. They just want to feel sorry for themselves over the strange FMS that has struck them down in their prime. Up to 30 percent of FMS patients have what is described as clinical depression and should be treated for that alone at the start.

One danger here is that when the depression continues for too long, it can aggravate the FMS. Depression can interfere with deep sleep, which makes several other fibromyalgia symptoms worse. Some doctors say that any level of depression should be treated if it lasts for more than six weeks.

There are other aspects of FMS that can cause depression. However here we're talking about the depression that happens just after the patient is correctly diagnosed as having FMS.

ACCEPTANCE

Acceptance is the final stage of the grief cycle. Slowly the FMS patient comes to realize what the situation is. Nothing is hopeless, and he hasn't a brain tumor or terminal cancer of some kind. She has fibromyalgia, which can be controlled and moderated and with a lot of work and struggle, she can live in almost the same fashion she did before. But it will take work. Now the patient is ready to understand the treatments and life style changes needed to cope with fibromyalgia.

BUILD A SUPPORT GROUP

Fibromyalgia isn't like double amputation—no one can see your illness or pain. This makes it even more important that you try never to feel that you are alone with your fatigue, your lack of sleep or your depression. You look healthy, you walk well, you can drive and go on trips. You don't look sick.

Sometimes when you tell friends about your illness they don't understand. Now, with more publicity and articles bout FMS, more people recognize the disease and what it entails.

Make a promise to yourself right here and right now, that you will never feel isolated and alone and unsupported. For a start, find someone you can talk to. If you have a spouse, that's the ideal solution. He or she knows of your pain and problems leading up to the diagnosis, and we hope has been with you all the way. If so, sit down and talk it out. Talk about the problems you need to work on right away, which ones you can put off, how you can get more deep sleep to help fix several things. We'll go into this area more later in the spouse section.

Just telling someone how you feel is going to do a lot to help you get through where you are now, and into your new phase of treatment and recovery.

Now, sometimes family members—even a spouse—will grow weary of the long diagnosis process. He or she isn't sure how to react when you don't know yourself what is wrong with you and how to fix it. Give it another try. Explain carefully that you have passed that stage, you are now diagnosed and treatment is being done right now, and that you hope for improvement.

The important element here is not to feel isolated, alone or stressed out. If so you can make many of your symptoms worse.

After you have your first confidant who you can talk to, branch out and develop a group of people you can rely on and talk to. In some places there are pre-organized support groups for FMS patients. Your doctor or a local hot line or the internet might be able to help you here. In such a group you'll hear the experiences of others who also have FMS and how they are coping. These groups can be of tremendous value, and it is a great idea to get your spouse to go along with you to the meetings.

Then on the way home you can talk about what you heard

and try to adapt the ideas or the methods into your own situation.

Another type of group you need is more a circle of friends than a group. These are people who believe in you, understand what fibromyalgia is and how it affects you. These people can be a tremendous help in day-to-day living. Say you don't have a car and you need to get to the doctor for your appointment. One of your friends may be able to drive you both ways.

Someone might come in once a week and help you with heavy cleaning that you simply can't do anymore. Maybe part of this group simply meets on Thursday noon for lunch at various local cafes and restaurants. The outing will do you good and you can order what you want—and what's healthy for you—and you don't have to cook or clean up. What a marvelous idea.

This circle of friends might come from other sources. If you work, there may be some there who will help you when they know of your situation. If you attend a church, chances are some friends there will lend a helping hand when you need one.

These people in your circle of friends do not have to be giving to you on a one-way basis. There might be something that you can do for them in return. Maybe you are staying at home now and could baby-sit for a neighbor's second or third grader after school until their mother gets home at 5:30. Don't do this for very small children or babies who are harder to care for.

Someone might have a dog you could board for a week while they are on vacation. There could be all sorts of services that you can offer to do for people who are helping you on an entirely different basis.

This sharing of help is the secret. Any time that one person is doing all the giving and the other getting all of it, the relationship is bound to break down. Think through what assets you have and what skills you can use in a turnabout sharing program with your friends and neighbors who are helping you.

For some people, it's hard to ask someone for help. In the supermarket it's easy: the box boy almost always asks if he can help you take your groceries to the car. Otherwise, it is harder.

Most of your friends, even the ones most sensitive to your special needs, won't be able to figure out all that you require in the way of help. It may be emotional need as well as physical. Just sitting with a friend over a decaf and talking about what is worrying you, or troubling you, is a help many of your friends can give. You ask them out for coffee. Pick up the tab and then bend their ears for an hour and a half.

THE SPOUSAL FACTOR

Every married woman who has FMS also has a spousal factor in her fibromyalgia equation. Yes, lots of men cut and run, and divorce a woman with FMS before either of them fully realizes what her sickness is.

For those who stick it out the factor becomes important. In the ideal situation, the spouse has been with the patient every step of the way from the first symptoms right through to the correct diagnosis of fibromyalgia. They have been through the pain and suffering and debilitating problems that severe cases can cause.

Now the two of them are in the treatment phase. This is good, and as it should be. Till death do us part, in sickness and in health, or something like this in the marriage vows.

The spouse who refuses to participate in the process—won't go with the patient to the doctor or take part in any of the support group activities—is only adding to the stress and problems of the patient. Such a spouse then becomes part of the painful problem of FMS, not a part of the solution.

The spouse should be tied into the treatment process as tightly as possible. Checking the daily pills, measuring medicine, checking routine and special appointments, helping evaluate sleep medications. Tracking sleep patterns and wakeful periods. Noting how many times the patient was awake during the night.

If the spouse can also participate in the stretching and exercising, so much the better. A two-mile walk will do the spouse good as well. Or let your spouse run out four miles, come back to the one-mile turnaround and then walk back home with you. There are all sorts of combinations of exercise and aerobic exercises that a couple can do together. It might be swimming, bicycling or hiking. At this point the more togetherness the better. It supports the patient. It gives the patient a feeling of being wanted and of being shown concern for the FMS problem and the ways to correct it.

Continual communication between the two of you is the most important element here. Talk it over. Talk about every aspect of your disease and treatment and ways to make things better. This must be an on-going dialogue to keep both of you up to date, and to be sure your spouse understands how you feel about everything. Don't shut each other out from any aspect of your medical or your emotional situation.

TO SEX OR NOT TO SEX?

Sexual intercourse has been described by experts as the best stress reliever possible. When pain is involved, sex becomes a dubious solution. It's something that both of you want, but when you try, it is frustrating, embarrassing and often unproductive.

Some FMS medications can sharply reduce sexual desire. Compound this with the situation where sexual activity becomes painful and so exhausting that it hardly seems worth the effort and you have real problems. Up jumps the psychological problem about how no-sex will affect the marriage. It's a real problem for many couples where one has FMS.

Yes, there are things you can do. The pain associated with sex may be an outgrowth of your general painful times in other parts of your body. Understand that proper sleep and other treatments can moderate your body pain. This then can reduce your pain when having sex.

Talk to your doctor about the problem. Granted, some doctors shy away from talk about sex. They shouldn't. Ask for medications that will not reduce your sexual desire. With a little experimentation you should be able to come up with the right ones.

Then, talk with your partner about the situation. Be assured that your spouse is still interested in your body, and that you can still turn each other on and be desirable. Sometimes this is part of the problem. You don't think you're so sexy any more. Not true. Despite your age—at least up to about 80—the two of you have grown older together. Whether it's ten years or forty, your sexual desires are still there. Dig them out.

Here are some other suggestions to help your sex life despite fibromyalgia:

If you are more vigorous and active in the morning, plan on having sex on a weekend morning. Work out some signals that you can give each other when you're thinking about sex. It might be a gentle massage of his shoulders, or running your hands through her hair. A gentle neck nuzzle or foot rub sends the right message.

If your medications affect your sex drive, adjust the time when you are planning sex. Take them after, not before. But take your pain medications so they will be strongest during your proposed sexual contact.

If you don't have a waterbed at home, find a motel that has one and reserve a room for that best time for you, and try out the waterbed. The rocking motion of the water is a real turn on for some people.

Talk during foreplay. Tell each other what excites you and what doesn't hurt. Let each other know your responses and ask for feedback. Couples who talk it out during sex often do much better than those who don't say a word.

If you plan on a sex time, try not to overtire yourself during the period before the appointment. You don't want to be tired and worn down.

Share a hot shower or bath before you get into bed. It can be a wild kind of foreplay that gets you both in the mood. The hot water will help moderate your pains as well.

Make your sexual positions the easiest and least strenuous. There are many books that can help you with positions. Also consider other means besides intercourse to gain sexual pleasure. Stimulating each other by hand to a climax is exciting for many.

Try some sexy music and a room full of lighted candles to get both of you in the right mood. This can work wonders. Remember, the experts say that good sex is only 40% physical—the rest is emotional.

Tell your partner where your sore muscles are and work around them. This is good to get out of the way before you undress so you don't have to talk about that in the middle of something wonderful.

Remember, orgasm isn't the only goal of good sex. You can thrill at the closeness of the other person, of the sexy massage, the sensual pleasure of being kissed all over your body. The lack of orgasm for either party, whether planned or accidental, should in no way be thought of as a sign of sexual failure.

MAKE EVERY DAY COUNT

A huge part of living with fibromyalgia is trying your best to make every day the best one yet. Yes, this is upbeat thinking—and it works so well it's a bit scary. Don't let your pains and your hurts and fatigue and all the rest of it get you down. Jump up and yell that it's a great day to be alive—because you still are.

That's reason enough to make this a day to be remembered. What can you do today to make it stand out? What can you do for someone else that they will remember and appreciate? People with FMS do a lot of receiving of help and encouragement. It's always a good time to do a little of the same thing for someone else who needs the help. It might be another FMS patient you know, or a stranger who needs a hand. Maybe a check sent to a family that was just burned out in a fire, or had a loved one killed and there's no money for a funeral. See how good your own life is?

Have you talked to yourself lately? Go ahead, admit it. We all do from time to time, at least in our heads. Sometimes we even get in arguments with ourselves.

Many times a lot of these unspoken arguments and words

can turn you either way. So make it a habit of talking good things and good plans and good deeds to be done. Think along these lines:

- I am living over and above my fibromyalgia, resolving to be strong and to be courageous in my outlook and activities.
- I can evaluate my FMS and get the treatment I need as I begin to take back my life almost the way it used to be.
- I know who I am, and I love that person, and accept myself for what I am, and know that I am improving all the time.
- I am more than capable of mastering this fibromyalgia disease and returning my body and mind to less pain, and know that I can live above and through this and the other symptoms.
- Yes, I have made mistakes, but from them I have learned and I have grown. Now I am not afraid to try new things, new medications, new ways of correcting the problems with my body.
- I am a person, a human being, what I am does not depend on what I can do physically. I am a mind and that mind has a body.
- I am no longer shy about asking for help when I need it. It helps me be stronger, and makes the day that I can be healthier and stronger still come that much sooner.

Today, and every day, I will concentrate on those things that I can do, and do well, and not worry about what is no longer possible for me.

KEEPING A JOURNAL

We mentioned before the idea of keeping a journal. Great idea. A journal is a record, and as such it can be a thousand different things and done a thousand different ways. One good thing it can do for you is to keep a record of your medications. By looking back in your journal you can tell what meds you were on, what strength, how many and when you took them. Any change in meds are shown and you may be able to regulate and figure out the med situation from your records.

Physically it can be anything. A school theme spiral bound booklet, or one with 200 pages. It can be a loose-leaf notebook. This is the one that works best for most people. If you use a computer to write your daily report, then all you have to do is three-hole punch the paper and put it in the notebook. This gives you an easy-to-read record and a convenient place to put the pages. Watch as the pages mount up.

You'll be interested to go back a year and see what you were writing about in your journal.

It's also a place for your small victories in any field, how you feel, where the hurts are, how the sleep project is coming along, what you did to dig out of your depression. Put it all down. It can help in more than one way. It's a record but it also is a kind of purging of your soul that is good for you.

Likes and dislikes can also go in here along with your dreams, your plans, even your romances. Get it all down and then see how interesting it will be in even six months.

So you don't forget to write your day's page—establish a set time to do it. This might be right after you eat dinner, or right before you go to bed. If you use a computer or typewriter, do a page of double spaced work. That's roughly 250 words and you can get a lot said in that space.

Try it, you'll be glad that you did.

THE EIGHT COMMANDMENTS

Thought there were ten? These are the eight commandments chiseled in the stone of your conscience to help you to make life easier for you as you live with your fibromyalgia. They are:

1. CUT AND SLICE

Take a look at your schedule. How many of the jobs and meetings and tasks on that list are essential to your life, your happiness and your sanity? Cut and slice and get rid of some of the things you may have been doing for years but don't really need to now—not with all the pains and fatigue you have now. If it isn't essential, cut it out.

2. ORGANIZE

Those things you have left to do should be set down in an orderly manner, economizing on time and travel. Plan any runs with the car you need to make so you can do several things at once instead of making two or three trips a day. Organize your daily tasks, your work projects—get more efficiency-minded.

3. TIME OUT

During the day be sure to build in a rest period. This might be right after lunch or right after dinner. Stretch out on your favorite couch or your bed, put a pillow under your head and close your eyes. A small snooze isn't out of place here. Do this consistently. But you'll never do it unless you organize it into your daily schedule.

4. ELUCIDATE

Be sure that your relatives and close friends understand what your disease is and how it saps your energy, disturbs your sleep, gives you major body pains and generally tries to shut you down. Tell them what you can and can't do these days, and promise them that you are working to get better so you can take on more tasks and more work projects. When they understand, they won't bombard you with all of the good work things you used to have time for—and that same person might even volunteer to give you a hand now and then.

5. KISS

That stands for Keep It Simple, Stupid. A fine idea. Try to make your life and your tasks as simple as possible. Someone said the simple way to do a job is the most efficient and the best way. Check over your must-do jobs and break them down into their most rudimentary elements. Then tackle them one at a time in sequence and life should move along a little smoother.

6. DELEGATE

When you have your schedule at the minimum and the tasks themselves cut to the simplest factors, you still may have more on your plate than is practical with your FMS. Delegate. Ask someone else to take over some of your traditional jobs.

You don't have to cook the turkey for the family gathering every Thanksgiving. You don't always have to host the Christmas party. Go to Uncle Joe's this year or Aunt Martha's house. Delegating saves your strength.

7. REMODEL

Look around your house or apartment. Are there things you could do with little work, or hire done, which would make your home so much easier to live in while you have FMS? Would a gentle wooden ramp up those three steps at the front door be a lot easier for you to walk up four or five times a day? Can your kitchen cabinets be lowered or restocked so the things you use are lower down? If you have a two-story house, should you move your bedroom to the ground floor until you are feeling better?

8. REEVALUATE

Step off the merrygoround of your life for a moment and reevaluate it. Are you doing some things you really can't physically do right? Are there some tasks you can do that you don't? What about that group you were going to join? Did you have that heart-to-heart talk with your spouse and your boss at work about your FMS and what you can and can't do? Reevaluate your life and try to find things you can change to make living better, more fun, and more fulfilling.

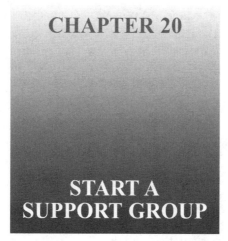

CHAPTER 20

START A SUPPORT GROUP

Y ou are not alone. Sometimes it might seem like it, but you are truly not alone in your battle with fibromyalgia. One of the best answers for your lonely feeling is to join a fibromyalgia support group. In most cities and larger towns you'll find one. This simply points out how many women and some men suffer from this condition.

How to find such a group? First talk to your doctor to see if he or she knows of an FMS support group in your area. Chances are there will be one. If your doctor doesn't know, phone other doctors who know about fibromyalgia and ask them. The next stop is to call your local hospitals and ask their community service managers if that hospital has such a group or if they know of any in your area.

Let's say you struck out. No such group in your area. So, your next job is to start a group yourself.

HOW TO START

It isn't as hard as it may sound. Go to the hospital you have used and ask them if they will help you form such a group and sponsor it. All they would have to do would be to provide you with a meeting room where you could meet once a month. Many hospitals will do this.

Let's say they agree. Your next step is to write letters to every national fibromyalgia organization you can find. We'll list three or four here. These groups come and go, some take new names and some simply run out of funds. Send the same letter to each of them telling them you're starting a support group for FMS and ask them for their expertise in how to go about it—and any printed material they can send to you that you can duplicate and use.

Here are some of the national FMS organizations.

American Fibromyalgia Syndrome Association
6380 E. Tanque Verde Road #D
Tucson, AZ 85715

Fibromyalgia Network
PO Box 31750
Tucson, AZ 85715-1750
Phone: 1-800-853-2929

Fibromyalgia Alliance of America
PO Box 21988
Columbus, OH 43221

Fibromyalgia Information Resources
PO Box 690402
San Antonio, TX 78269

One of these sources will be able to help you, and you might get good information from all of them.

Now, what else can you do?

You might also find out the phone number of the Arthritis Foundation chapter in your state. Since the problems are much the same, they sometimes have material they can give you to help form your group.

TALK TO YOUR DOCTOR

Your doctor probably treats other patients with fibromyalgia.

He can't give you their names or phone numbers, but go prepared to give him a dozen or so sheets of paper with your name, address and phone number on it, and ask that they be given to any patients he thinks a support group might help. Most doctors are glad to do this—but usually it's the nurses who get the job done.

MAKING GOOD MEETINGS

Now you have a start. Talk to your contact at the hospital where they are loaning you a free meeting room. Ask if you can put up a notice about a meeting on their bulletin board. Some hospitals have them and some don't.

It might be helpful to put a small advertisement in the daily paper under personals: "Wanted, Fibromyalgia patients who would like to form a self-support group. I have FMS too, so call me at 000-1010 and let's talk." Such an ad run in the Friday, Saturday and Sunday newspaper might produce some good leads.

Even before your first meeting, you can distribute flyers about it at area libraries, physician's offices, osteopaths, rheumatologists, and other heath professionals who have contacts with fibromyalgia patients. Ask them to put one on their bulletin board, or give copies to patients who have FMS. Every little bit helps.

Some newspapers, TV and radio stations have places where they announce community meetings and events. Try to get your session posted there every time you meet. This can reach a huge audience, depending on the size city you are in. The best part, this is free as a community service.

As the meeting approaches, you should have received material from some of the national associations. Look it over and decide what would be good to duplicate to give to each person at the meeting.

If you don't feel ready to chair the group or to lead the meeting, find one of your friends or new acquaintances who will do the job. It's not that complicated. You show up at the meeting place, welcome those who come, chat for a while and then at or near the appointed time, get the people's attention and get the meeting going. One of the first things to do is to pass a clipboard around with paper and pen on it and ask the people to sign in with their name, address and telephone number.

You will probably want to tell the people there who you are and why you decided to start a support group and then explain what you hope to do. You might include:

1. Open by telling who you are and that you have FMS. Tell a little about your problems, main concerns, and why you started the group.
2. Then go around the room and have all present introduce themselves and tell a little about their situation.
3. Have an open forum for talk about FMS.
4. Let people tell their experiences, and report any success with some type of treatment.
5. Have a time for questions by the participants with the hope one of the people can offer some answers or some support.
6. Suggest early on that there will be no bad mouthing any doctors or health groups. Keep everything positive.
7. Make clear that anything said in the group, stays within the group. Everything said at these meetings is strictly confidential, and must not go beyond the four walls. The only exception might be to use information to be of help or assistance to someone who needs it.
8. This is a support group. No criticizing nor judging is allowed. This is a support group, not a judge or a jury.
   After you've been meeting for a time, new people will come. That's great. You may want to have a newcomer packet, explaining the group, what you do, how you try to help. You may also want to take the person aside and explain in person the guidelines about sharing and confidentiality, and how you are all victims and hoping to get better.
9. Let the people suggest what they want to do at the meetings and what they hope to get out of them.

10. See if anyone has any helpful hints how to cope with FMS at home, at the office or when traveling. You'll be surprised at the good ideas many of the women will come up with.
11. Ask the group if this is a good time to meet.
12. Ask if they want to meet once a month or more often.
13. Ask if they want to have medical specialists to come talk to them about FMS.
14. Ask if they know of anyone else who has FMS and might be benefited by the group.
15. Urge the people to bring a new person to the next meeting.
16. Ask if anyone has trouble with transportation and see if anyone lives near those people who could offer a ride.
17. Set the time and date and place for the next meeting, and urge all to come.
18. Ask for a volunteer to be telephone contact to call each of the people the week before the next meeting to remind them to come.
19. Thank everyone for coming and tell them you look forward to the next meeting where more of you can share your experiences.

SPEAKERS

Who might be asked to speak to your group? Doctors, pharmacists, rheumatologists, nurses with special FMS interest—any health-oriented person who has something to say to help you.

You might find someone who could be of use to those in the work place, where education is needed for management. Soon you should set up a person to be in charge of speakers to contact and book these people.

Some groups send out mail notices. Some groups have a small membership fee to cover the cost of mailing. (20 letters, 12 times a year at .33 = $79.20.) No one member should have to contribute the cost of postage and Xeroxing…(20 x .05 x 12 = $12.00). This part of your group might come a few months after you get moving.

Speakers should not take up the whole meeting. This is a support group as well as educational. Members will find release and relief when they can tell about some particularly trying situation or type of pain or depression that they have been through. Others listening may be able to gain some insight and benefit from what any member says. Always allow at least half of the meeting for the members to talk. After the formal meeting is over, there may be time for networking and talking with others and with the speakers on a one-to-one basis.

SLOW START?

Your group may get off to a slow start. If you have friends or know of others who have FMS be sure to get them to come to the first meeting even if you have to drive over and pick them up. You could have only three or four at a first support group meeting.

Don't worry about it. Talk with each other and get a start on trading aches and pains and cures. Then for the next meeting ask those there to bring a friend who has FMS, or a caregiver. Then redouble your efforts at getting the word out about the support group.

If there's a local group specializing in arthritis, it may have some names of members of that support group who have FMS and go there since there wasn't one specifically for them. Now there is. Get their names or have the other group notify them about your meeting.

Talk with your doctor again. Tell her of your first meeting and urge her to let patients know about it. Doctors understand how such groups can support patients. Most doctors who treat FMS patients will be glad to help you find new members.

EXPANDING THINGS

As your group grows, you'll need help to keep it moving. Ask people to take on responsibilities. Make out a list of committees needed and ask for volunteers. Look for people to take on:
  • Membership mailing notices.

- Finding speakers
- Telephone contact to take calls from the flyers for new members.
- Posting flyers in various public service bulletin boards, the TV station, radio and newspapers.
- Setting up refreshments and cleaning up.
- Obtaining books and literature about FMS and making material available to the group.

SUPPORT FOR YOUR GROUP

In come cases a hospital will sponsor your group by making available a meeting room and sometimes coffee as well. Contact the local chapter of the Arthritis Foundation. The state group or the national one often will sponsor an FMS group since it is so close to the arthritis syndrome. They sometimes make available training for the group leader, and provide sample press releases, mailing expenses, lists of speakers available, and literature on FMS.

In some cases the Fibromyalgia Network—address above—will send free information about starting a support group. This group also has a subscription newsletter that should be worth investigating.

So, there you have it. Enough information and addresses to get you off and running to form an FMS group. Try to get another person to co-chair this with you from the git-go. Then it won't be so lonely out there—or exhausting—before you get your group going.

Good luck!

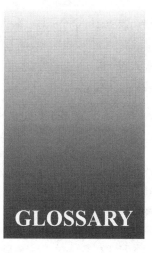

GLOSSARY

ACETAMINOPHEN: A fever reducing and pain relieving non-prescription, over-the-counter product.

ACUPUNCTURE: An old Chinese healing art that inserts extremely thin pins into specific points of the body to relieve pain.

ACUPRESSURE: The use of pressure over specific muscles to relieve pain and aid healing.

ACUTE: Pain that begins quickly, is sharp or severe and intense.

AEROBIC: Activities that create increased oxygen consumption by the body, such as walking, running, or swimming.

ANEMIA: A condition when the body has fewer than normal red cells in the blood.

ANTIBODY: A blood protein made by the body in response to a foreign substance. An antibody binds to an antigen and eliminates it from the body.

ANTIDEPRESSANT: A medication utilized in relief of depression or the blues. Tricyclic antidepressants help to relieve night-time muscle spasms in fibromyalgia patients.

ANTIGEN: Any substance the body thinks is foreign or potentially dangerous, that results in the production of an antibody.

ANTIHISTAMINE: This medication inhibits or counteracts the action of histamine, a biological chemical produced in an immune response. Histamine dilates blood vessels and stimulates the secretion of gastric juices. Antihistamines can cause drowsiness—a problem for fibromyalgia patients with stress and fatigue.

ANTI-INFLAMMATORY DRUG: A drug (including ibuprofen and aspirin) which reduces redness, swelling, heat and pain.

APNEA: The hesitation or stopping of breathing during sleep caused by obstruction within the nasal airway. Can happen a number of times during the night.

ARTHROSCOPIC SURGERY: Surgery done on a joint or tendon using a small flexible tube inserted through a small incision.

ATROPHY: When an organ, tissue or muscle decreases in size, usually through disuse.

AUTOIMMUNE DISEASE: A problem created by the action of the immune system working against itself because the immune system can't tell the body's own tissue from foreign elements.

BIOFEEDBACK: A way of utilizing equipment to monitor the heart rate, skin temperature, muscle tension and blood pressure. These readings show on a monitor so people can see how their bodies react to stress or pain, so they can learn how to control their own responses.

BIOLOGICAL: A laboratory product similar to the body's own bio-chemicals, and which—when given as a drug—alters the body's immune response.

CARTILAGE: A smooth tough fiber that covers the ends of the bones so they don't rub directly against each other.

CHROMOSOME: The basic structure in the nucleus of every cell containing genetic material that determines the cells' individual characteristics.

CHRONIC: Persisting for a long period of time.

CHRONIC FATIGUE SYNDROME: CFS. A condition that produces fatigue on a long term basis. The symptoms are nearly identical to FMS except for the intense pain with fibromyalgia.

COMPLETE BLOOD COUNT: A test that measures all components of the blood, including numbers of white and red cells and platelets.

CAT Scan: Computerized Axial Tomographic scan. A special X-ray that produces thin cross sectional images of the body.

Connective Tissue: Long fiber body tissue that supports and connects internal organs, forms bones and walls of blood vessels, attaches bones to muscles, and replaces tissue following surgery.

Corticosteroids: Hormones produced by the body related to cortisone. They can be synthetically produced and have powerful anti-inflammatory effects. Prednisone and cortisone are such drugs available by prescription.

Cortisone: Potent steroid drug that reduces swelling and inflammation, but can have serious side effects.

Deep Heat: Tissue penetrating ultra-sound waves to heat up small portions of the body and penetrate deep into the tissue.

Delta Sleep: This is deep, restorative and replenishing sleep required for the vital functions of the body including antibody production and immune functioning. Delta waves are brain waves produced by this deep sleep.

Depression: That state of mind producing feelings of worthlessness, irritability, lack of sleep, anxiety, dejection and low self-esteem.

Fibromyalgia: A syndrome of musculoskeletal pain, stiffness, chronic aching, and tenderness of certain sites. This condition is so named when not associated with other diseases or conditions such as cancer, thyroid disease or rheumatic arthritis.

Flare Up: A time when symptoms worsen or increase in severity.

Genetic Markers: Specific genes, or groups of genes on individual chromosomes that indicate a genetic tendency, including that for developing certain diseases.

Hemoglobin: A protein that moves oxygen through the blood.

Ibuprofen: A nonsterodial and anti-inflammatory drug available over-the-counter.

INFLAMMATION: The body's protective response to injury or infection. Heat, redness, swelling and pain result from a biochemical secretion that comes from the immune cells as they fight the problem.

LIGAMENT: A tough cord-like fiber that attaches to the bones to keep the bones in correct alignment.

MRI: Magnetic Resonance Imaging. A magnetic picture of body parts and soft tissue that won't show up on an X-ray. It is non-invasive like an X-ray.

METABOLISM: How the body uses food to produce energy and build new body tissue. It breaks down the food into energy. This affects the metabolic rate and the number of calories used in an hour.

NITRATES: A food preservative found in cured meats that may cause joint swelling in some people.

NSAIDs: Nonsterodial Anti-Inflammatory Drugs. These are a group of drugs with fever-reducing and pain-reducing effects because they can stop the synthesis of prostaglandins. These include ibuprofen, aspirin and many prescription drugs.

PLACEBO: An inert substance in pill or injection form, administered under the guise of effective medication. May also be used in controlled and double blind clinical testing. About 20% of people using a placebo will show improvement. This is purely psychological in nature and called the "placebo response."

PSYCHOLOGIST: A non-medical person schooled in psychology who is licensed to offer practical advice of a therapeutic nature. A psychologist can't prescribe drugs.

REMISSION: The cessation or slowing of symptoms of a disease.

TENDON: A strong band of tissue that connects muscle to bone.

TENDINITIS/TENDONITIS: Soreness and inflammation of a tendon.

ULTRASOUND: A technique using sound waves to reveal deep structures of the body on a screen which then can be recorded on a video or printed out on paper.

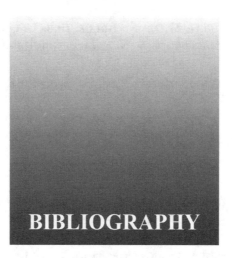

BIBLIOGRAPHY

COPELAND, MARY ELLEN, *The Depression Workbook*, Oakland, CA, New Harbinger Publications, 1992.

CONLEY, DR. EDWARD J., *America Exhausted*, Flint, Michigan, Vitality Press, 1997, 1999.

CATALANO, ELLEN M., *Getting to Sleep*, Oakland, CA, New Harbinger Publications, 1990.

ELROD, DR. JOE M., *Reversing Fibromyalgia*, Pleasant Grove, Utah, Woodland Publishing, 1997.

Fibromyalgia Syndrome and Chronic Fatigue Syndrome in Young People, Tucson, AZ, Fibromyalgia Network.

FRANSEN, JENNY, RN, & RUSSELL, I. JOHN, M.D. PH.D., *The Fibromyalgia Help Book*, Saint Paul, MN, Smith House Press, 1996.

GARDISER, KIT, ED., *We Laughed, We Cried, Life With Fibromyalgia*, Palo Alto, CA, KMK Associates, 1995.

GOLDBERG, BURTON, *Chronic Fatigue, Fibromyalgia & Environmental Illness*, Tiburon, CA., Future Medicine Publishing, 1998.

KHALSA, DHARMA SING, M.D., *The Pain Cure*, New York, Warner Books, 1999.

LEWIS, KATHLEEN, *Successful Living With Chronic Illness*, Dubuque, IA, Kendall Hunt Publishing, 1995, 1997.

McIlwain, Harris H. M.D., and Bruce, Debra Fulghum, *Fibromyalgia Handbook*, New York, Henry Holt & Co., 1996, 1999.

Pellegrino, Mark J, *Fibromyalgia, Managing the Pain*, Columbus, OH, Anadem Publishing, 1993.

Powell, Robin I., *The Working Woman's Guide to Managing Stress*, Englewood Cliffs, NJ, Prentice Hall, 1994.

Register, Cheri, *Living With Chronic Illness*, New York, Bantam Books, 1987.

St. Amand, R. Paul, M.D. and Marek, Claudia Craig, *What Your Doctor May Not Tell You About Fibromyalgia*, New York, Warner Books, 1999.

Starlanyl, Devin, M.D. and Copeland, Mary Ellen, M.S., M.A., *Fibromyalgia & Chronic Myofascial Pain Syndrome*, Oakland, CA, New Harbinger Publications, Inc., 1996.

Starlanyl, Devin, M.D., *The Fibromyalgia Advocate*, Oakland, CA, New Harbinger Publications, Inc., 1999.

Van Why , Richard, *Fibromyalgia Syndrome and Massage Therapy*, Frederick, NM, Richard van Why Publishing, 1994.

Williamson, Miryam Ehrlich, *The Fibromyalgia Relief Book*, New York, Walker and Company, 1998.

Williamson, Miryam Ehrlich, *Fibromyalgia, a Comprehensive Approach*, New York, Walker and Company, 1996.

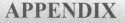

APPENDIX

FAT GRAMS PER SERVING CHART

The foods in the following table are listed in category alphabetically. They are listed by food group, not as "apple" but apple is shown under fruit. Some products are listed by themselves, but all are in categories such as: bread, cakes, eggs, margarine, pasta.

Since many of us are also interested in the calorie count on food, I'll also list the calories for each serving.

Note: "T" in the fat grams column means "trace."

FOOD	SERVING	FAT	CALS
BACON			
Armour Star, cooked	1 slice	3	38
Oscar Mayer, cooked	1 slice	3	35
Nathan's Beef Bacon	3 slices	7	100
BEEF			
Tenderloin	3 oz	12	208
Top round	3 oz	8	170
Top sirloin, fried	3 oz	19	277
BEER			
Schlitz	12 oz	0	145
Miller Lite	12 oz	0	96
BREAD			
Weight Watcher's Cinnamon Raisin	1 slice	T	60
Pepperidge Farms	1 slice	3	90
Wonder, Wheat	1 slice	0	70
Light Oatmeal	1 slice	0	45
Pita, whole wheat	1 oz	1	80
Roman Meal	1 slice	1	68
French bread	1 slice	1	100
BUTTER			
Cabot	1 tsp	4	35
Land O'Lakes	1 tsp	4	35
Land O'Lakes Whip	1 tsp	3	25
CAKE MIXES			
Angel food	1/12 cake	0	150
Banana cake	1/12 cake	11	250
Carrot cake	1/12 cake	15	232
Chocolate w/frosting	1/8 cake	17	300
Date quick bread	1/12 loaf	21	60

FOOD	SERVING	FAT	CALS
CHICKEN			
Breast quarters w/skin	1 oz	2	42
Breast quarters skinless	1 oz	T	31
Leg quarters w/skin	1 oz	4	49
Dark meat batter dip	5.9 oz	31	497
Dark meat, roasted	3.5 oz	16	256
Banquet Fried Chicken	6.4 oz	19	330
Swanson Fried Chicken	4.5 oz	20	360
CHILI			
Chef Boyardee Chili Con Carne w/ Beans	7 oz	20	340
Dennison's Chili w/Beans	7.5 oz	19	300
Van Camp's Chili w/Beans	1 cup	23	352
Health Valley Vegetarian	5 oz	3	160
POTATO CHIPS			
Eagle Chips	1 oz	10	150
Kelly's Rippled	1 oz	9	150
Lance Rippled	1 oz	13	160
Pringle's Chips	1 oz	13	170
Weight Watchers BBQ	1 oz	6	140
COFFEE			
Instant regular, black	6 oz	0	4
Regular brewed, black	6 oz	0	4
COOKIES, READY TO EAT			
Nabisco Raisin Oatmeal	1	3	70
Angel Bars	1	5	74
Lance Apple Oatmeal	1.65 oz	7	190
Anisette Toast Jumbo	1	1	90
Chips Ahoy Choc-Walnut	1	6	100
Nutra/Balance Choc Chip	2 oz	14	260
Lance Choc-O-Mint	25 oz	10	180

Fat Grams Chart

Food	Amount	Fat (g)	Calories
Lemon cake, frosting	1/8 cake	17	300
Crumb coffeecake	1/6 cake	7	230
CANDY			
Almond Joy	1.76 oz	14	250
Butterfinger	2.1 oz	12	280
Hershey w/Almonds	1.45 oz	14	240
Lifesavers	1 candy	0	40
M & M Peanuts	1.7 oz	13	250
Mr. GoodBar	1.7 oz	19	290
Gum drops	1 oz	0	100
CEREALS (WITH 1/2 CUP 1% MILK)			
Alpha Bits	1 cup	1.5	212
100 % Bran	1/3 cup	3.5	170
Apple Raisin Crisp	2/3 cup	1.5	230
Bran Flakes	1 oz	2.5	200
Ralston Rice Chex	1 cup	1.5	194
Froot Loops	1 cup	2.5	210
Corn flakes	1 cup	1.5	210
Quaker Life	2/3 cup	3.5	200
Quaker 100% Natural	1/4 cup	7.5	227
Cream of Wheat	1 oz	2.5	208
Instant oatmeal	1 cup	3.5	245
CHEESE			
Blue cheese	1 oz	8	100
Brie	1 oz	8	95
Armour Cheddar	1 oz	9	110
Bristol Gold Lite	1 oz	4	70
Colby	1 oz	9	110
Edam	1 oz	8	100
Kraft Gouda	1 oz	9	110
Monterey Jack	1 oz	9	110
Swiss	1 oz	8	110
Heath Valley Apple Spice	3	T	75
Tastykake Fudge Bar	1	8	240
Frookie Ginger Spice	1	2	45
Sunshine Lemon Coolers	2	2	60
COTTAGE CHEESE			
Borden 5% Dry Curd	1/2 cup	1	80
Knudsen 2%	4 oz	2	100
Land O'Lakes	4 oz	5	120
Weight Watchers 1%	1/2 cup	1	90
CRACKERS			
Nabisco Cracked Wheat	4	4	70
Goya Butter Crackers	1	1	40
Cheese crackers w/Peanut butter	1.4 oz	11	210
Cheez-it	1	2	470
Dark Rye Crisp Bread	1	T	26
Nabisco Escort	3	4	70
Keebler Garlic Melba toast	2	T	25
Saltines	2	1	25
FROZEN DINNERS			
Armour Classic Chick/ Noodles	11 oz	7	230
Armour Lite Chicken Ala King	11 oz	7	290
Banquet Chicken Nuggets	6 oz	16	340
Budget Gourmet Chicken Caccitori	1 pkg.	27	470
Budget Gourmet Lite Pot Roast	1 pkg.	8	210
Le Menu Beef Stroganoff	10 oz	24	430
Le Menu Lite Glazed Chicken	10 oz	3	230
Lean Cuisine Fillet Fish	10 oz	5	210
Swanson Chicken Nuggets	9 oz	23	470

FOOD	SERVING	FAT	CALS
Weight Watchers Baked Fish	7 oz	4	150
DOUGHNUTS			
Tastykake Chocolate Dipped	1	10	181
Earth Grains Devil's Food	1	21	330
Powdered sugar minis	1	3	58
Tastykake Fudge Iced	1	21	350
Glazed donuts	1	13	235
EGGS			
Fried with margarine	1	7	91
Hard boiled	1	5	77
Scrambled	1	7	101
Egg white only	1	0	17
One egg yolk poached	1	5	59
Egg Beaters (substitute)	1/4 cup	0	25
Scramblers (substitute)	3.5 oz	5	105
FISH			
Smelt	6 oz	6	212
Red snapper	6 oz	3	217
Microwave tuna sandwich		6	200
Rainbow trout broiled	3 oz	4	129
Canned tuna in water	3 oz	2	90
Canned tuna in oil	3 oz	15	200
S&W canned tuna in water	3 oz	1.5	90
Orange ruffy baked	3 oz	1	75
Sea bass, broiled	3 oz	2	105
Groton's Frozen Scrod	1 pkg.	18	320
Van Kamp's Frozen Fillets	1	10	180
Mrs. Paul's Fish Cakes	2	7	190
Microwave Fish Sandwich	1	15	280

FOOD	SERVING	FAT	CALS
HAMBURGER			
Double patty w/bun	1 reg.	28	544
Double patty, all fixings	1 reg.	32	576
Double patty, all fixings	1 large	44	706
Single patty, w/bun	1 reg.	12	275
Single patty, bun, cheese	1 reg.	15	320
Single patty, all fixings	1 large	48	745
Triple patty, all fixings	1 large	51	769
HOT DOGS			
CHICKEN:			
Health Valley	1	8	96
Weaver	1	10	115
TURKEY:			
Bil Mar Cheese Franks	1	9	109
Louis Rich	1	9	103
Mr. Turkey Franks	1	11	132
Wampler Longacre	1	31	102
BEEF:			
Armour Star Jumbo	1	18	170
Hebrew National	1	15	160
Oscar Mayer Bun Lengths	1	17	186
Oscar Mayer Wieners Little	1	328	
ICE CREAM, ICE DESSERTS			
Bresler's All Flavors Ice	3.5 oz	0	120
Bresler's Ice Cream	3.5 oz	12	230
Edy's light Almond Praline	4 oz	5	140
Sealtest Butter Crunch	1/2 cup	9	160
Lady Borden Butter Pecan	1/2 cup	12	180
Haagen-Daz Chocolate	4 oz	17	270
Weight Watchers Ice Milk	1/2 cup	4	120
Ben & Jerry's Chocolate Fudge	4 oz	16	280

FRUIT

Item	Serving	Fat (g)	Calories
Fresh apple	1	T	81
Fresh grapefruit	1/2	0	40
Dry, pitted prunes	1/4 cup	1	140
Fresh orange	1	T	69
Fresh pear	1	1	100
Fresh pineapple	1 cup	1	90
Canned mixed fruit	1/2 cup	0	90

* Most fresh fruits have almost no grams of fat. Canned fruits have little more, but the sugar content raises the calorie count.

FRENCH TOAST

Item	Serving	Fat (g)	Calories
Home-made w/egg, milk	1 slice	7	155
Take-out, with butter	1 slice	9	180
Aunt Jemima Cinnamon Swirls	3 oz	4	71
Weight Watchers French Toast	2 slices	5	160

GELATIN

Item	Serving	Fat (g)	Calories
Royal Apple	1/2 cup	0	80
Jell-O Black Raspberry	1/2 cup	T	81
Cherry w/Nutrasweet	1/2 cup	T	8
Diamond Crystal Orange, sugar-free	1/2 cup	T	9

GRAVY (CANNED)

Item	Serving	Fat (g)	Calories
Franco-American Beef	2 oz	1	25
Franco-American Pork	2 oz	3	40
Pepperidge Farm Beef	2 oz	2.5	65

HAM

Item	Serving	Fat (g)	Calories
Armour Star Boneless	1 oz	2	41
Hansel 'n Gretel Deluxe	1 oz	1	31
Krakus Polish cooked	1 oz	3	65
Oscar Mayer Cracked Black	1 oz	T	24
Russer Lill' Salt cooked	1 oz	1	30
Canned extra lean	1 oz	2	41

Item	Serving	Fat (g)	Calories
Good Humor Chocolate Malt	3 oz	13	187
Weight Watchers Treat Bar	2.75 oz	0	90
Breyers Coffee Ice Cream	1/2 cup	8	150
Mocha Mix Dutch Chocolate	3.5 oz	12	210
Land O'Lakes Fruit Sherbet	4 oz	2	130
Wyler's Fruit Punch Slush	4 oz	0	140
Ben & Jerry's Health Bar	4 oz	17	300
Jell-O Orange Bars	1	T	42
Borden Orange Sherbet	1/2 cup	1	110

JAMS, JELLIES

Item	Serving	Fat (g)	Calories
Smucker's Fruit Spreads	1 tsp	0	16
Pritikin Fruit Spreads	1 tsp	0	14
White House Apple Butter	1 oz	0	50
Bama Grape Jelly	2 tsp	0	25
Apple Jelly	3.5 oz	0	259
Strawberry Jam	3.5 oz	0	234
Plum Jam	3.5 oz	0	241

* No jams, jellies, fruit preserves, etc. contain fat.

LUNCHEON COLD CUTS

Item	Serving	Fat (g)	Calories
Armour Bologna Beef	1 oz	8	90
Carl Buddig Pastrami	1 oz	2	40
Hansel 'N Gretel Healthy Deli Bologna Beef & Pork	1 oz	2	41
Oscar Mayer Bologna	1 slice	8	90
Oscar Mayer Honey Loaf	1 slice	1	35
Weight Watchers Bologna	1 slice	1	18
Hard Pork Salami	1 slice	4	41
Summer Sausage Thuringer	1 oz	8	98

MARGARINE

Item	Serving	Fat (g)	Calories
Fleischmann's Diet	1 tbsp	6	50
Mazola Diet	1 tbsp	6	50
Parkay Diet Soft	1 tbsp	6	50

FOOD	SERVING	FAT	CALS
Smart Beat	1 tbsp	3	25
REGULAR STICK:			
Blue Bonnet	1 tbsp	11	100
Fleischmann's	1 tbsp	11	100
Land O'Lakes	1 tbsp	4	35
Mazola	1 tbsp	11	100
Parkay	1 tbsp	11	100
SOFT TUB:			
Blue Bonnet	1 tbsp	11	100
Fleischmann's	1 tbsp	11	00
Land O'Lakes Tub	1 tbsp	4	35
Parkway Soft	1 tbsp	11	100
Promise	1 tbsp	10	90
Parkay Whipped	1 tbsp	7	70
MAYONNAISE			
Low Calorie:			
Best Foods Cholesterol Free	1 tbsp	5	50
Best Foods Light	1 tbsp	5	50
Kraft Free	1 tbsp	0	12
Kraft Light	1 tbsp	5	50
Smart Beat Corn Oil	1 tbsp	4	40
REGULAR:			
Best Foods Real	1 tbsp	11	100
Hellmann's Real	1 tbsp	11	100
Kraft Real	1 tbsp	2	100
Sandwich Spread	1 tbsp	5	60
MEXICAN FOOD FROZEN			
Banquet Chimichanga	9.5 oz	21	480
Banquet Enchilada Cheese	11 oz	9	340
El Charrito Burrito Grande	6 oz	16	430
Enchilada Cheese Dinner	14 oz	24	570

FOOD	SERVING	FAT	CALS
2% milk	1/2 cup	2.5	60
Buttermilk	1/2 cup	2	60
Whole milk regular	1/2 cup	4	75
Skim milk	1/2 cup	T	45
NUTS			
Cashews, peanuts	1 oz	12	170
Planters Mixed, Salted	1 oz	15	170
Guy's Tasty Mix	1 oz	7	130
Dry roasted w/peanuts	1 oz	15	169
Planters' Almonds	1 oz	15	170
Black Walnuts	1 oz	17	180
English Walnut halves	1 oz	20	190
Cashews	1 oz	14	170
Cashews dry roasted	1 oz	13	163
Filberts	1 oz	19	191
Peanuts dry roasted	1 oz	14	170
Peanut butter	2 tbsp	17	200
Pecans	1 oz	20	190
COOKING OIL			
Crisco	1 tbsp	14	120
Planter's Popcorn Oil	1 tbsp	13	120
Puritan	1 tbsp	14	120
Wesson Corn	1 tbsp	14	120
Smart Beat	1 tbsp	14	120
Wesson Vegetable	1 tbsp	14	120
Crisco Solid	1 tbsp	12	110
Wesson Shortening	1 tbsp	12	100
ORIENTAL FOODS (FROZEN)			
Benihana Lites Chicken	9 oz	42	70
Birds Eye Stir Fry Vegetables	1/2 cup	T	36

Food	Amount	Fat	Calories
Corn tortillas	2	1	95
Healthy Choice Enchiladas	13 oz	5	350
Healthy Choice Fajitas	7 oz	4	210
Lean Cuisine Enchanadas	10 oz	9	290
Patio Enchilada Beef Dinner	13 oz	24	520
Patio Fiesta Dinner	12 oz	20	460
Van De Kamp's Beef Burrito	5	9	320
Van De Kamp's Mexican Classics:			
Chicken Suiza w/Rice, Beans	15 oz	20	550
Enchilada Suiza Chicken	5.5 oz	10	220
Weight Watchers Fajitas	7 oz	5	210
Taco shells	1	2	50

MUFFINS

FROZEN:

Food	Amount	Fat	Calories
Sara Lee Apple Oat Bran	1	6	190
Health Valley Banana Free	1	T	130
Sara Lee Blueberry	1	8	200
Sara Lee Blueberry Free	1	0	120
Pepperidge Farm Cinnamon Swirl	1	6	190
Sara Lee Golden Corn	1	13	240
Health Valley Oat Bran	1	4	140

MUFFIN BOX MIX:

Food	Amount	Fat	Calories
Arrowhead Blue Corn	1	4	110
Duncan Hines Bran, Honey	1	4	120
Duncan Hines Cran-nut	1	8	200
Duncan Hines Wild Blueberry	1	3	110

MILK

Food	Amount	Fat	Calories
Evaporated	1/2 cup	10	170
Evaporated Skim	1/2 cup	0	100
Carnation dry milk	8 oz	T	90
1% milk	1/2 cup	1.5	51

Food	Amount	Fat	Calories
Birds Eye Chow Mein	1/2 cup	4	89
Chung King Walnut Chicken	13 oz	5	310
Chung King Egg Rolls Shrimp	3.6 oz	6	200
La Choy Pork Egg Roll	3 oz	5	150

TAKE OUT

Food	Amount	Fat	Calories
Chicken teriyaki	3/4 cup	27	399
Chop suey with pork	1 cup	24	425

PANCAKES AND WAFFLES

Food	Amount	Fat	Calories
Hungry Jack Blueberry	3 4-inch	15	320
Aunt Jemima Buckwheat	3 4-inch	8	230
Hungry Jack Buttermilk	3 4-inch	11	240
Hungry Jack Packets	3 4-inch	3	180
Arrowhead Griddle Lite	1/2 cup	3	260
Estee Pancake Mix	3 3-inch	0	100
Pancakes with butter, syrup	3 4-inch	14	519

PASTA

* Most pastas are 1 gram of fat per 2 oz. The differential here is what is put in the pasta or on it. Calories for plain pasta range from 160 per 2 oz to 210.

Food	Amount	Fat	Calories
Dry pasta, all types	2 oz	1	210

PASTA DINNERS, FROZEN:

Food	Amount	Fat	Calories
Banquet entree Primavera	7 oz	3	140
Banquet Macaroni & Cheese	7 oz	11	260
Budget Gourmet Stroganoff	1 pkg	12	290
Budget Gourmet Cheese Manicotti	1 pkg	25	430
Dining Light Fettuccini	9 oz	12	290
Green Giant Cheese Tortellini	1 pkg	9	260
Healthy Choice Fettuccini	8.5 oz	4	240
Kid Cuisine Macaroni, Franks	9 oz	15	360
Le Menu Light Tortellini	8 oz	8	250
Lean Cuisine Rigatoni, Meat	10 oz	10	260

FOOD	SERVING	FAT	CALS
Morton Macaroni & Cheese	6.5 oz	14	290
Swanson Spaghetti and Meat Balls	13 oz	18	490
Weight Watchers Manicotti	10 oz	8	260

PICKLES

☆ All cucumber pickles have either 0 grams of fat or a trace.

PIE

Frozen:

Banquet Apple	1 slice	11	250
Sara Lee Apple	1 slice	12	280
Mrs. Smith's Apple Natural	1 slice	22	420
Banquet Banana	1 slice	10	180
Mrs. Smith's Blueberry	1 slice	17	380
Banquet Lemon	1 slice	9	170
Banquet Pumpkin	1 slice	8	200

BAKED READY TO EAT:

Apple	1 slice	18	405
Creme	1 slice	23	455
Lemon meringue	1 slice	14	355

PIZZA, FROZEN

Celeste Deluxe	8 oz	32	600
Fox Deluxe Sausage	1/2 pizza	13	260
Jeno's 4 Pack Cheese	1 pizza	8	160
Jeno's Crisp Sausage	1/2 pizza	16	300
Pappalo's French Pepperoni	1 pizza	20	410
Totino's Bacon Party	1/2 pizza	20	370
Totino's Mexican Style	1/2 pizza	21	380
Weight Watcher's Cheese	7 oz	7	300

POPCORN

Jiffy Pop Microwave Butter	4 cups	7	140
Newman's Microwave Light	3 cups	3	90

Calories vary but go from a low of a trace in diet drinks to 190. Most are about 75 or 80 calories. No big worry about fat grams from soft drinks.

FOOD	SERVING	FAT	CALS
TURKEY			
FRESH:			
Louis Rich Breast	1 oz	2	50
Perdue Breast Fillets	1 oz	T	28
Louis Rich Breast Steaks	1 oz	T	40
Perdue Fresh Drumsticks	1 oz	2	36
Bill Mar Ground Turkey	3 oz	12	163
Louis Rich Thighs	1 oz	4	65
Shady Brook Wings	3 oz	6	130
Whole Turkey	3.5 oz	10	200
SOUP			
CANNED:			
Healthy Choice Bean & Ham	7.5 oz	4	220
Campbell Bean w/Bacon	8 oz	4	140
College Inn Beef Broth	7 oz	0	16
Campbell Beef Noodle	8 oz	3	70
Lipton Beef Noodle	8 oz	T	85
Goya Black Bean	7.5 oz	4	160
Gold's Borscht	8 oz	0	100
Health Valley Chicken Broth	7.5 oz	2	35
Campbell Chicken Corn Chowder	11 oz	21	340
Pritikin Lentil	7 oz	0	100
Snow's Clam Chowder	7.5 oz	2	70
Health Valley Minestrone	7.5 oz	3	130
American New England Chowder	4 oz	6	145
Pritikin Split Pea	7.5 oz	T	130
Campbell Tomato w/2% milk	8 oz	2	90
Campbell Vegetable	8 oz	2	90

Item	Serving	Fat (g)	Calories
Redenbacher Gourmet			
Original	3 cups	4	80
Pillsbury Microwave Butter	3 cups	13	210
Ultra Slim-Fast Lite	1/2 oz	2	60
Weight Watcher's Ready Eat	.7 oz	3	90

SALAD DRESSING

READY TO USE:

Item	Serving	Fat (g)	Calories
Catalina	1 tbsp	1	15
Diamond Crystal Blue Cheese	1 tbsp	1	20
Kraft Bacon & Tomato	1 tbsp	7	70
Kraft Free Catalina Nonfat	1 tbsp	0	20
Ott's Italian Chef	1 tbsp	9	80
Newman's Olive Oil and Vinegar	1 tbsp	9	80
Seven Seas Free Ranch Nonfat	1 tbsp	0	16

READY TO USE LITE:

Item	Serving	Fat (g)	Calories
Estee Blue Cheese	1 tbsp	T	8
Herb Magic Vinaigrette	1 tbsp	0	6
Kraft FrenchMagic Mountain	1 tbsp	1	20
Blue Cheese	1 tbsp	T	5
S&W Italian No Oil	1 tbsp	0	2
Ultra Slim-Fast	1 tbsp	T	6
Weight Watcher's Russian	1 tbsp	5	50

SAUSAGE

Item	Serving	Fat (g)	Calories
Oscar Mayer Bratwurst, Smoked	2.7 oz	21	237
Perdue Turkey Patties	1.3 oz	4	61
Armour Country Sausage	1 oz	11	110
Hebrew National Knockwurst	3 oz	25	260
Oscar Mayer Polish	2.7 oz	20	229
Armour Link Pork Sausage	1 oz	11	110
Perdue Sweet Italian Turkey	2 oz	6	94

SODA DRINKS

* All but four of the popular soft drinks now on the market have no fat grams at all. Of the four that do, two are root beer, one a ginger ale and the other a wild berry.

VEGETABLES

MIXED, FROZEN:

Item	Serving	Fat (g)	Calories
Hanover broccoli, cauliflower	1/2 cup	0	20
Broccoli, cauliflower, carrots w/cheese sauce	1/2 cup	6	89
Chinese stir fry	1/2 cup	T	36
Japanese stir fry	1/2 cup	T	29
Mixed vegetables w/onion	1/3 cup	5	97
Oriental blend	1/2 cup	0	25
Peas, onions, cheese sauce	1/2 cup	6	126
Stew vegetables	3 oz	T	50
Peas & onions cooked	1/2 cup	T	40
Fresh zucchini	1/2 oz	T	3
Canned tomatoes	1/2 cup	T	40
Canned spinach	1/2 cup	0	25
Fresh shallots, chopped	1 tbsp	T	7
Sauerkraut, canned	1/2 cup	0	20
Fresh baked potato	5 oz	T	220
Canned peas	1/2 cup	0	90
Canned corn	1/2 cup	0	70
Canned carrots	1/2 cup	0	20

YOGURT

Item	Serving	Fat (g)	Calories
Cabot all flavors	8 oz	3	220
Apples 'N Spice No-fat	8 oz	T	190
Black Cherry Classic	8 oz	6	230
Colombo Blueberry Classic	8 oz	6	230
Dannon Blueberry No-fat	8 oz	0	100
Yoplait Blueberry Original	6 oz	3	190
Knudsen Lemon w/Aspartame	6 oz	0	70
La Yogurt Peach	6 oz	T	190
Mountain High Plain	8 oz	9	200
Meadow Gold Raspberry Sundae	8 oz	4	250
New Country Strawberry	6 oz	2	150

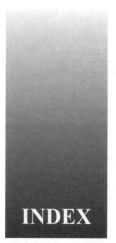

INDEX